Global Reset

Health, Wealth, Coincidence and
the Covid-19 Pandemic

Thomas A. Smith

Published in 2020 by FeedARead.com Publishing

Copyright © Thomas A. Smith.

First Edition

The author has asserted their moral right under the

Copyright, Designs and Patents Act, 1988, to be identified

as the author of this work.

A CIP catalogue record for this title is available from the
British Library.

To all those underpaid health workers who provide care to anyone who needs it.

Table of Contents

List of Figures

Preface

This book came together during the 2020 Covid-19 pandemic, while I was confined to my home not far from Mulhouse and close to the heart of the French epidemic. The pandemic crystallised a project that had been long in gestation and was originally intended as a leisurely undertaking for when I was retired.

Since I am an infectious disease epidemiologist by profession, the reader may wonder how I could have written this I should have been out in cyberspace fighting the pandemic. In fact, my day job of trying to stem infectious disease was precisely what made this possible. Initially, I did not get involved with models of Covid-19, or with the public debate, partly because one voice is easily diluted out, and partly because I was not an expert on respiratory viruses. In parallel with working with colleagues on how to try to avert catastrophic consequences of the breakdown of health systems in Africa, we were also adapting our public health teaching to make it more immediately relevant (by including Covid-19 examples) and moving it onto an online platform we had not used before. There were plenty of other people modelling Covid-19, and I was hoping that my three-and-a-half decades spent researching and teaching in health statistics and infectious disease modelling have contributed some relevant skills to those who are working with health agencies to mitigate the pandemic. But, as a disease modeller I saw little point in trying to add more admissions of uncertainty into the cacophony in the public sphere (a theme elaborated on in Chapter 9135) [1], where sound advice was mixing promiscuously with lies and confusion. Half the population of the world seem to have re-invented themselves as experts on the epidemiology of Covid-19.

Within a few weeks my reticence about getting directly involved in modelling of Covid-19 had been swept aside by demands to engage with policymakers in formulating the Swiss policy. When hard data became available about what was happening, it became possible to contribute usefully in ways that were previously unimaginable. The initial involvement with the team advising the Swiss health authorities, stimulated me to add to my notes on the themes of these essays. Writing became my escape from an overload of professional demands and hubbub of news about the pandemic. At a certain point though it made sense for younger colleagues to take over the high pressure demands for frequent updates of analyses and detailed advice on policy, and I concentrated on completing these essays.

This book is aimed at the general reader, rather than at any specific discipline, and it does not apologise for being a work of advocacy; I would be flattered if you find that it has made you think or changed your opinions. It is written from a public health point of view as a wide-ranging critique of the role of economics in our society. It is also, in places, a light hearted story (with some cheeky asides) about an imaginary being (economic man) falling sick and dying; or it is just a set of essays on topics that happen to be related to each other, laced with a few personal anecdotes. Obviously, had I set out calmly to write a book aspiring to be just one of these things, I would have focussed it on just one of them, but that was not where my mind took me. The pandemic resonated with many themes that I had been thinking about for decades, and during sleepless nights, writing this served as an alternative to stressing-out colleagues with complicated emails while they were trying to juggle unreasonable professional demands with living in confined spaces. I am tremendously fortunate in sharing a spacious home and a large garden with a loving partner who tolerates a degree of craziness.

I am one of those over-60s classified as having an underlying condition and hence considered in an at-risk group. Members of that age group should also feel a sense of responsibility for having propagated the other disasters that this book refers to[2]. We should have some humility when asking younger generations to look after us.

Only a few weeks ago we were following the sailing-boat voyage of Greta Thunberg across the Atlantic, struggling to undo the damage that my generation has inflicted on the world. Events since then have proven wrong the naysayers who think that nothing can change the trajectory of our civilisation. Today Thunberg's voyage would be impossible. This is a critical time when the future of our world is uncertain, and this will provide myriad opportunities to turn it in new directions, either insidious or wonderful. We need to make sure that business-as-usual is a thing of the past.

My training is in the natural sciences and statistics, so probably scientists and statisticians (especially Bayesians) may find my argument and writing style most accessible.

Finally, I would like to acknowledge the colleagues and friends who found time to give feedback on this manuscript, despite the stress we are all living through. It is meant as opinion, intended to be provocative, and you were not expected to agree with it all. I hope you do not mind seeing your names in the acknowledgements[3]. Some parts of it will no doubt be downright wrong. Maybe we can work together on an improved second edition. Marina Antillon, Günther Fink, Monica Golumbeanu, Julie Telford, Nakul Chitnis, Gail Smith, Chris Weeks, Don de Savigny, Derek Charlwood, Liz Erett, Sylvia Gray, Roger Harmon, Joanna Schellenberg, Sara Randall, Anne Gray, Sue Johnston-Wilder, Aatreyee Das, Katya Galactionova, Allan Schapira, Mark Blaxter, Mark Lambiris, Josh Yukich, Rebecca Lawson. Special thanks to Lars Kamber for assistance with graphics.

To the reader seeking entertainment I offer a quote from the Austrian novelist Thomas Bernhard "*There is nothing to praise, nothing to condemn, nothing to incriminate, but there is much that is ridiculous; it is all ridiculous, when you think of death.*"[4]

1   The Centre for Evidence Based Medicine needed until early April 2020 to assemble a meta-analysis of all the mathematical models that were being developed[1]. Why do so many modellers think it is useful to reinvent disease models rather than to build on what others have already done?

2   To avoid misunderstanding at the start, I insert a spoiler here by stating that this book is not about blaming the pandemic on ecological imbalances.

3   I should acknowledge a conflict of interest in that I receive funding from the Bill and Melinda Gates Foundation, and wrote this in Microsoft Word on a Windows 10 computer. This may or may not have influenced comments I make about Bill and Melinda. In case either of them ever reads this, I assure them that I did not use their funding to support writing this book (so I am not going to mention the grant number). If I reassigned any time that I was meant to be working on malaria to something else, it was to the work on the Covid-19 pandemic. I also hope this does not offend colleagues who think Word is rubbish. I could not have written this book using any other software.

4   Original: "*es ist nichts zu loben, nichts zu verdammen, nichts anzuklagen, aber es ist vieles lächerlich; es ist alles lächerlich, wenn man an den Tod denkt.*"

Introduction

"Health is the most important end of development as well as the most important means."— Amartya Sen[1]

This book began as a set of essays about health and wealth and turned into an extended argument that health considerations should be at the heart of decision making, where all too often they are absent. Life is a precondition for everything else and good health is one of our most basic needs[2]. Though it is not the only thing that matters to us[2], we value health both for its own sake and because without it, everything else we value generally becomes much more difficult.

While health often appears as a footnote in political and economic plans, economic arrangements are often presented as having inherent importance. Various orthodoxies in economics have dominated policy making in the western world to varying extents since the industrial revolution, mostly giving people the impression that we are trapped in a world of inequality and anxiety. But the economic arrangements we have are just one contingent set of ways of doing things that has been created to organise production and distribution.

The world we live in is permeated with quirkiness and chance, which profoundly affects the ways people behave, our social structures, and our health[3]. The role of luck, both good and bad, undermines grand theories of everything, including those in the field of economics.[4] The Covid-19 pandemic illustrates this with many examples of chance phenomena. It also injects an urgency into the need to agitate for fundamental changes to the *status quo* of recent public policy, because the randomness makes it possible for all kinds of things to happen in the wake of the pandemic[5]. Much more is at stake than just the final size of the pandemic. Various ideologies perpetrated by economists of one kind or another account for many of the other challenges we face. While this is the first economic crisis since World War II where the cause is not economic, it is also likely to provide the best opportunity to put these dogmas in their places, before they lead us into further, far worse crises.

To place this argument in context this book starts with a condensed history and pre-history of health and wealth (Chapter 1). This excursion in the fields of economic pre-history and anthropology is there to provide background on what it means to be human, but the pre- history began even before there were humans, with the biology of our primate ancestors so there is also some evolutionary biology here.

In the centuries since Hobbes[3] and Rousseau[4] first speculated about an original state of nature[6], much has been learnt about the intertwined histories of health and wealth. We have lots of data (but also many uncertainties) about how hominins became human and then transformed themselves into the clients of today's consumer capitalism, worrying about their health insurance. Health was always an issue for our ancestors, as was the acquisition of resources and overcoming scarcity.

Chapter 2 moves the history forward into the contemporary world, showing that on key measures of health, life-expectancy and avoiding epidemic disease, there has been enormous progress since the industrial revolution. The perception that this history is over is illusory. The Covid-19 pandemic is a unique event, only in the sense that every major event is unique. This implies a much broader agenda than just ensuring the adequacy of health services, because health depends on risk factors of many different kinds (including psychosocial factors as in status syndrome [5], and the effects of economic inequality[6]), and on preventative interventions. These are discussed in Chapter 3.

Trading in markets dates back only a few thousand years. Chapter 4 explores how one highly influential school of econometrics does or does not fit in to this history. Instead of explaining actual economies, the standard economic model plays a strange quasi-religious role operating in a theoretical world in which some neat mathematics applies. The philosopher Plato would have approved[7]. He believed that there are two realms or levels of reality, the everyday world, and that of eternal forms. His ideal society is ruled by philosopher kings. The high priests of the

Chicago School of Economics would also agree. They have wielded tremendous influence linked to the invention of some of the mathematics. Sometimes the remoteness of their theories from the messy world inhabited by chance events is not obvious. A mathematical model divorced from reality can include randomness (something which is particularly relevant to epidemics and elimination of infectious disease)[7], but that is not the same as making it depend on data from the real world like most natural science.

To choose an example outside a narrow definition of health: economics does not tell us how much oil is in the ground (which is a geological question), or whether it should stay there (a question framed here as a matter of well-being). Its role should be to design institutional arrangements to make sure that it stays there, if that is what human well-being requires. One way of thinking about this is to follow Noah Yoval Harari[9] in classifying the world into natural phenomena and fictions, which include institutional arrangements and economic organisation. This makes it possible to understand that it is not economic arrangements that fundamentally limit human possibilities, that the distribution of wealth and income is something that is decided collectively by humans, some of them having more say than others, and that therefore it can be changed.

After this break from the dense non-fiction that makes up most of this book, Chapter 5 returns to earth with a discussion of how the primacy of economic ideology distorts international development, and sometimes makes it difficult for people working in public health to be clear about what they are doing, and why.

Progress happens despite this confusion, and Chapter 6 is a brief overview of one specific example, that of insecticide treated nets (ITNs) against malaria, where insights and approaches from the natural sciences and from economics have usefully come together to deliver enormous health benefits to some of the poorest and most marginalised people on the planet. This is an area of good news in the last decade[10], defying the sense of doom and gloom that has overshadowed much of the West.

Hovering in the background of this, like the grim reaper, is the question of the value of life. Some economists and decision theorists have taken upon themselves the role of working out what humans value and use this to claim a special status in providing inputs to policy decisions. Chapter 7 is a discussion of rational choice theory, the basis of much of health economics, and of its limitations. This critique largely aligns with the capabilities approach associated with the philosopher Martha Nussbaum, and the development economist Amartya Sen. Sen won the Nobel Memorial Prize in Economic Sciences in 1998 for his criticisms of rational choice theory, and his proposal for an alternative, placing health at the centre of decision making, (but recognising that it is not the only thing that matters). 'Health' should in any case be understood as a shortened version of 'health and well-being' with caring for our environment[8] as part of caring for human wellbeing[9]. The pandemic provides an in-your-face example of where conventional economics has collided with the prioritisation of health. The lockdowns and the repurposing of economies around the provision of ventilators and diagnostic tests could never have happened if governments had stuck to the rules of economic advisors.

Chance and quirkiness are everywhere and It is easy to think of the Covid-19 pandemic as either an anomalous black swan event[12][10] with no implications other than that we should try to get back to normal as soon as possible afterwards; or as the realisation of the Coming Plague, predicted by Laurie Garrett two decades ago[13]; or the first of a series of horses-of-the-apocalypse linked to our abuse of Gaia[11]. Without screening newspaper articles and blog posts to work out which of these interpretations is currently more popular, but none of these models really fit the facts of what is happening now.

There is nothing inevitable about the economic system we had until last month, and the temporary domination of policy making by one strange set of models of the economy may eventually seem like an aberration resulting from some chance events in the intellectual history of the 19th century. In political terms the claims of this book amount to an assertion that economics should be subsidiary to health and wellbeing, i.e. the health people should be calling the shots. This requires us to separate the tasks of analysing what is physically and humanly possible (the role of empiricist science); the identification of what economic arrangements are needed to facilitate the health outcomes that we want (the legitimate role of economics); and democratic politics. The latter is ultimately where the responsibility lies for making the challenging decisions about life and death that cannot be avoided when different policy options lead to trade-offs between morbidity states and life or death of different people. It is quite feasible to separate out the value-laden elements of decisions about health, from analyses of what are the likely consequences of different options.

This needs to be understood more broadly than a proposal to put the Ministry of Health in charge of economics[12]. That would be a challenge: many of the finest analytical minds that should have been working out how to improve our health, have spent the last few decades in the finance sector competing with each other for who can cream off the most resources from everybody else. At a time when health budgets across the world average just over 9% of government expenditure[14] it might seem to be a utopian prospect for health to be prioritised over the perceived interests of the extreme rich. Except that this is what happened in March 2020 almost everywhere. The dog has finally begun to disobediently wag its tail. The details of the current arrangements though, are not exactly ideal, and no-one knows what will happen next.

To make sense of our world, we humans habitually arrange our thoughts as stories[15]. One story that is familiar to me as a public health professional is the human life history. I have structured this book as a life history of capitalism. You may think you can guess the ending. If so, good luck!

---

1   The quotations in the chapter headings of this book are not intended as axioms or articles of faith. They should be read as thought-provoking statements made by others that relate to the topic of the chapter.

2   The concept of health here is one that has evolved from that in the original constitution of the World Health Organisation written in 1946, which states that 'health is a state of complete physical, mental and social well-being and not merely the absence of disease or infirmity'. 'Health' should thus be understood as a shortened version of 'health and well-being' with caring for our environment as part of caring for human wellbeing. There are many other things that we value, like a healthy environment, fairness, freedom of thought and expression, and good relationships with those around us.

3   The first draft of this book started with a chapter arguing that nature is everywhere permeated with randomness. Many people find that argument hard to accept. It is easy to believe that for practical purposes we should attribute much of what we experience to chance, irrespective of whether nature is deterministic or stochastic.

4   It also contradicts the dogma of classical Marxism, the ideology used by the Communist regimes that competed with capitalism during the 20th century. Communists claimed that the victory of the workers was inevitable (at least until it became obvious that it wasn't). In which case, why did so many people in the 20th century sacrifice their lives on the altar of Leninism? Why move your arse if you can rely on the implacable advance of the forces of history? The hardliners could handle this because they liked contradictions. (Geneva used to have a similar problem with Calvinists).

5   Technically randomness is not the same as mathematical chaos, but from a practical point of view it may appear similar.

6   Debates about whether humans are fundamentally peaceful as asserted by Rousseau, or violent (Hobbes) are often framed in terms of the contrast between these two philosophers, both of whom were speculating wildly since they had negligible archaeological and anthropological evidence to go on. Chapter 1 argues that humans began neither in an anarchist utopia, nor a chaotic bloodbath.

7   Mathematical models are descriptions of systems using mathematical terms. Some include assumptions about how real-world data are distributed around the quantities of interest and are used for estimation. These are statistical models. Others don't require any real-world data. They can nevertheless be stochastic (i.e. include effects of chance) if they assume that the system itself is inherently random. Conversely deterministic models are those that assume that the system is not random. If this is not confusing enough, nowadays it is possible to fit stochastic models to data, usually using Bayesian Markov Chain Monte Carlo methods[8]. Many practitioners are themselves confused about these distinctions (and therefore don't necessarily distinguish stochastic and statistical models in this way). Many don't realise that they are doing something very different from other 'modellers'.

8	Important questions need to be settled about how to address the climate emergency, but time has been wasted because public policy has been dominated by the absurd dogma that economic growth should be its primary objective (Chapter 5). In principle competition for resources between humans and other organisms is unavoidable because we are all part of the natural world, but the sun provides far more energy than we use. I suspect that the exit strategy from the climate emergency may be to directly harness solar energy with technologies that cut out our dependence on photosynthesis[11]. We should concentrate ourselves in cities and allow rural areas to rewild. Others may believe that we should all eat only organic vegetables and try to be self-sufficient.

9	There are unanswered questions about other issues like animal rights here, but let's also leave worrying about dogs and cats until after the pandemic is over.

10	'Black swan' events are rare and unpredictable outlier events that may have big effects. If you have never seen a black swan you probably think they are all white. Taleb was a stock-market trader obviously inspired by market crashes, but these are perhaps not the best example since they only appear extremely rare to a young person considering a limited time horizon.

11   When the pandemic began there were green politicians aghast that it would distract attention from the climate emergency, only for it to become obvious a few days later that it would produce a wealth of evidence to further their cause. The pictures of nature in the Venice lagoon, and the twittering birds in our garden, serve as compelling experimental evidence of the benefits of decarbonising our lifestyles. There is a philosophical issue about whether we care about the natural environment for its own sake or our own. In the universe there are vast numbers of inaccessible planets with interesting things on them. I don't think very many humans care when an astronomer reports that a galaxy somewhere has just exploded. We are only interested in the planet we live on because it is the one inhabited by humans.

12   This would be unimaginable in Switzerland, because of the decentralisation of the health system and the weakness of the federal health ministry, even compared with other federal government departments.

1. From Conception to Adolescence: Prehistory and History of Health and Wealth

"..... when the woman saw that the tree was good for food, and that it was a delight to the eyes, and that the tree was to be desired to make one wise, she took of the fruit thereof, and did eat; and she gave also unto her husband with her, and he did eat." —Genesis 3 v6.

The myth of the Garden of Eden describes God's original sin against humanity, Eve is depicted weighing up nutritional, aesthetic, and intellectual considerations, against the injunction of the patriarch to leave Him to make His own incomprehensible and arbitrary decisions. The subsequent mess was documented in the Torah/Old Testament, and turned into films by Hollywood, where the patriarchal values seem to have rubbed off on some of the studio directors. A lot of plagues and massacres might have been avoided had Eve been left to make the decisions in a responsible way, taking these various aspects into account.

According to one religious cult, invented in the 16th century by a crazy guru in Geneva, and transmitted around Europe in the form of an outbreak called the Reformation, God also came up with the work ethic (for details see [16]) and it is commonplace for economists to tell as 'there is no such thing as a free lunch'. That there is no way of getting something for nothing. In a seemingly sterile city environment, lined with asphalt, concrete, and shops and restaurants it may seem obvious that they are right. Humans, the argument goes, have always needed to work for their sustenance.

Try telling this to the birds and the bees! Animals do not work for their food, they forage. They need to expend energy to do this, and there are many trade-offs embedded by evolution in the possibilities they have for exploiting their food supplies. We are primates, and other primates are also foragers. Primates are an exceptional group of organisms in the diversity of their behavioural/life strategies, which involve adapting to different environments, especially the things they do to obtain mates. Different species have different mating systems and patterns of aggression and domination. Some of them form life-long pairs, others are promiscuous, like bonobos; some of live in polygamous groups dominated by aggressive males. These mating strategies and patterns of dominance and submission of different species can be related to availability of food and foraging strategies.

Often the behavioural pattern of an animal changes over time, for instance most mammals have defined breeding seasons, and are not interested in sex the rest of the time. The physiology and behaviour of male gorillas changes dramatically if they achieve dominance. All this is driven by switching of hormonal systems, which, like much in biology are messy, difficult to understand, and often have unanticipated consequences.

We are interested in primate behaviour because there are obvious similarities between humans and other primates, but unlike a typical monkey species which can generally be characterised by a limited set of foraging strategies, humans have a varied repertoire of life strategies. The biology of human behaviour appears to be a wonderful mess. Not only do people vary in their mating strategies, dominance relationships, and ways of getting resources, but we may change our strategies from time to time, rather unpredictably. The human brain has an extraordinary plasticity[17], and some humans, like virtuoso violinists, or Olympic athletes make extraordinary achievements that others can only marvel at, by specialising in specific skills.

Until agriculture began with the Neolithic revolution[1], humans foraged. The anthropologist Marshall Sahlins used examples from around the world to show that gatherer-hunters don't need to work especially hard for their lunch[19]. Sahlins quotes Eyres[20] description of human foraging.[2] There were decisions to be made about whether to go hunting for mammoths (or outsize kangaroos) or to pick berries, but there was no trading going on in the sense we understand it nowadays. The idea that gatherer-hunters were busily bartering mammoth meat for blackberries as early adopters of the division of labour as

-15-

described by Adam Smith[21], is a myth [22]. Of course, there was division of labour within family groups. No doubt the men thought themselves superior because occasionally they brought down an item of megafauna[3] but the women probably did most of the work involved in putting something to eat on the pile of stones in the middle of the cave.

This depiction of an idyllic state of nature misses out the times when the water dried up, or the places that looked promising for fishing proved barren. Just like the animals that we may watch on nature videos, people helped themselves to food when it was available, and starved when it was not. There was no police force. Strangers were a threat, leading to pre-emptive violence, which could escalate into simmering tribal warfare[23]. Scarcity was always around the corner. On average these people did not live very long.

Remnant gatherer-hunter populations like the Hagahai in Papua New Guinea, the Yanomami in the Amazon, or the San people of the Kalahari, live in marginal environments where survival might be expected to be even poorer than that of most of our ancestors. In the mid-1980s, my colleague the anthropologist Carol Jenkins found that in the Hagahai, living in the remote fringes of the New Guinea Highlands 568 out of every 1000 infants died before their first birthday[24]. This may be an extreme case, compounded by the effects of infectious diseases introduced by outsiders. More usually, about 20% of gatherer-hunter children died before their first birthday [25], and up to half died in childhood, mostly of infectious disease. Those who survived this often lived into their 60s, so that on average such people lived about 30 years (see explanation of life expectancy in Chapter 8).

There is a widespread myth that market economies arose from barter systems in such societies, but in stone-age cultures, like those in PNG only a century ago, neither barter nor money was very important[22]. There is a substantial anthropological literature describing how exchange in such societies was via gifts. A seminal document in this field is the survey of gift exchange across the world, by Marcel Mauss[26], and an often-cited example is the 'big man' culture of the New Guinea Highlands.

Because of the warm, wet climate in New Guinea, the staple foods there are root crops, food storage is almost impossible without a refrigerator, or a pig. In highland areas pigs fed on sweet potatoes were the main store of wealth. Power and influence were gained by throwing a party (or mumu), where large numbers of pigs were killed and cooked in earth ovens[4]. The invitees would feel beholden to the host and throw their own parties. The one who could throw the biggest party would gain respect and influence over the others, allowing him to accumulate more pigs.

In such gift exchange systems power and influence are gained by destroying wealth (i.e. pigs) in mumus, rather than by accumulating it. This system only works up to the scale of a couple of hundred people where everybody knows everybody else. Beyond that, our brains cannot cope with the size of the social network[27]. This is roughly the size of a New Guinea village, perhaps explaining why large-scale hierarchical societies never developed there.

A variant on this way of achieving wealth and power is cargo cult, where the cult leader convinces his followers that performing a specific ritual would make goods appear out of nowhere[5]. A famous example was the John Frum cult on the island of Tanna in Vanuatu[28]. After the US servicemen left at the end of World War 2, the followers of this cult built symbolic air strips and marched up and down, anticipating that this would induce planes to land and bring a cornucopia of goodies.

Power and influence still operate along similar lines in Papua New Guinea[6], and archaeological evidence suggests that such arrangements based on gift exchange (or hopes of gift exchange) were widespread until the spread of grain-based agriculture which originated in the Asiatic mainland. Reading Mauss'[26] and Sahlins'[19] descriptions of the nuances of different systems of kinship, reciprocity and exchange in traditional cultures (almost all of which have now vanished) it might seem that this is all a thing of the deep past. But kinship means family, reciprocity and gift exchange are what Christmas presents are about[7]. A moment's thought about how we have reacted in these times of crisis reminds us that gift exchange systems are still a big part of our lives, but they completely fail to conform to the principles of the rational choice or management theory, (though they remain very much a part of the practice of effective management[8]).

Although our brains still contain a lot of interesting stuff derived from primate biology and pre-history, political and economic arrangements did not start their lockdown until the rise of cities and the agricultural revolution. Hierarchical states are generally thought to have arisen in early agricultural societies in the river valleys of Asia, because of the need to store grain during the winter and drought periods (i.e. scarcity)[30, 31]. Whoever controlled the granaries could set themselves up as the king[9]. These cities seized control of the areas around them, and brutally employed forced labour to maintain their food production, trashing the pre-existing systems of kinship and reciprocity. Life expectancy is thought to have fallen below that of gatherer-hunters at some stages of early agriculture[25]. It was also these early states that introduced money, and linked to it, trading in markets[22].

The first documented epidemics (those in the Book of Exodus), were the diseases of crowding, mostly zoonoses (diseases originating in animals like Covid-19) which took hold in these cities when they reached a certain size[10]. As empires came and went in the ancient world, there was an overall trend for the largest centres of population to grow, and hence to become vulnerable to novel pathogens. As each new disease arrived in human populations with no immunity there was a series of massive epidemics[32]. 20th and 21st century scholars have debated which one corresponded to which of the pathogens we recognise today.

Angus Deaton summarised the history of wellbeing and survival from the beginning of agriculture until the enlightenment period as one of broadly stable life expectancy, and slowly growing population[25] but to the people living through this it must have very much depended on the chance event of when you were born. To school children learning about significant events in history, it might appear that there was just a sequence of famines, epidemics and wars. At times it must have seemed that everything was up in the air, and nothing could be relied upon, death and destruction was all around. But just as there is a cognitive bias in thinking change was gradual, there is a cognitive bias in thinking that crisis was the norm. Epidemics and wars take up a disproportionate amount of space in the history books relative to their extent in time. Similarly, military structures figure disproportionately in remains from the past, because they were built more solidly than anything else. For instance, there was a boom in castle-building in France in the 12th century CE and then again in the Vauban period 500 years later.[11]

Most of the evidence that we have for the health and survival of individual people prior to the 17th century is from skeletal remains (for instance the age distribution of the skeletons in cemeteries)[12]. Life expectancy at birth averaged only about 30 years throughout most of this period. There were many generations of people who did not experience dramatic upheavals, and very likely had the impression that their own uneventful lives were typical, and that their descendants would have similar lives to their own.

But these peaceful interludes were not an equilibrium where nothing was changing. From one generation to the next, there was accumulation of the debilitating twins of debt[13] and inequality[22, 34]. Inequality fell dramatically only (or at least mainly) in crisis situations associated with extreme violence or disease. During periods of feudalism-as-usual it gradually increased.

This phase of human history more or less corresponds to the almost two millennia required for the diseases of Asia, Europe and Africa to spread across this large, contiguous land mass, as described in the chapter headed 'Confluence of the Civilized Disease Pools of Eurasia: 500 BCE to 1200 CE' In William McNeill's history of the spread of infectious disease around the world[32]. Not so long after this phase ended, there was possibly the most spectacular recorded epidemic in Europe, the Black Death or bubonic Plague of 1348-9. Some historians believe that the economic dislocation that followed from this initiated the series of events leading to the industrial revolution. It disrupted the *status quo* primarily by creating labour shortages, increasing the bargaining power of workers leading to real wage increase. This could only happen because there were massive decreases in population.

But this was not accompanied by any general improvement in health. Plague epidemics came and went for the following 400 years[14]. Some of these epidemics also led to massive destruction of capital, which reduced the political power of owners and financiers. When the next big crisis occurred in the first half of the seventeenth century, life expectancy was still somewhere close to a value of 30 years even in the good years without wars and plague, just as it had been for millennia. Then the Reformation, one of the last eruptions of the medieval plague bacterium *Yersinia pestis,* and the 30-years war[15] (1619-48)[35] all coincided. Estimates of the proportion of the population killed by this war and plague are impossible to disentangle, because the armies were responsible for much of the spread of *Yersinia,* and half the population would have died in the course of this period, even without the crisis. Wilson claims the war killed a quarter of the population of central Europe[35], but a more accurate statement would perhaps be that few people who were alive at the start, were still alive at the end. Those inclined to see the current Covid-19 pandemic in an apocalyptic light, might find solace in this comparison, unless they happen to be living in a care-home.

The early seventeenth-century mortality in Europe was perhaps not even especially high in comparison to that experienced by the people of the Americas and the Pacific islands, when the Eurasian and African diseases, especially smallpox and influenza, were introduced round about the same time[32]. In post-Columbian Mexico it is generally estimated that more than half the population died [34], but further north mortality may have been even higher and it seems possible that entire civilisations were wiped out in the Amazon basin.

---

1   Recently there have been suggestions that the beginning of agriculture is better described as a gradual process with scattered evidence of domesticated plants and livestock going back as far as 9000 BCE, rather than an abrupt revolution, but that does not affect this argument. Walled, territorial statelets began about 3100 BCE [18].

2   "Throughout the greater portion of New Holland, where there do not happen to be European settlers, and invariably when fresh water can be permanently procured upon the surface, the native experiences no difficulty whatever in procuring food in abundance all the year round. It is true that the character of this diet varies with the changing seasons, and the formation of the country he inhabits; but it rarely happens that any season of the year, or any description of country does not yield him both animal and vegetable food....Of these [chief] articles [of food], many are not only procurable in abundance, but in such vast quantities at the proper seasons, as to afford for a considerable length of time an ample means of subsistence to many hundreds of natives congregated at one place.... On many parts of the coast, and in the large inland rivers, fish are obtained of a very fine description......"

3   Probably a species that is remembered now only in myths about dragons.

4   Mumus are not very hygienic (personally I tried to avoid eating the pork when attending mumus when we lived in PNG). Because the traditional diet between mumus consists of little more than sweet potatoes, mumus can result in large outbreaks a disease called 'pigbel' caused by the bacterium *Clostridium perfringens* and associated with spikes in protein intake against a normal diet very low in protein. Pigbel was almost eliminated by vaccination but in recent years is returning because vaccine production ceased as a result of cost-cutting.

5   Nowadays this sometimes works, if the ritual entails sending an application to the Bill & Melinda Gates Foundation.

6   When archaeologists painstakingly excavate Neolithic settlements in Europe and try to interpret what they find in order to understand what was going on ten thousand years ago. I am reminded of when we lived in PNG in the 1980s and would take visitors for a walk in the bush, pointing the ruins of Neolithic villages. These were probably about 20 years old. They were the places where the people had been living for defensive reasons before the Australian colonial administration's attempt to suppress tribal warfare.

7   Christmas stirs up many conflicting emotions because its origin in multiple pre-Christian Roman festivals, some involving gift exchange and some not, and its history of takeovers by Christianity and consumer capitalism[29], mean that many people feel torn or confused about it, as witnessed by all the broken resolutions not to give any presents this year. Although it accounts for a substantial proportion of consumer expenditure in the industrialised world, something less likely to make sense in terms of rational choice theory (Chapter 7) is hard to imagine.

8   For some reason, Mauss did n7ot consider gift exchange in industrialised societies. We pretend it is not important, but for a long time I reported to someone who operated very effectively this way. I am not sure if he is aware of the deep anthropological roots of this management technique, or that anyone in his staff might be aware of the literature on the topic. So long as it worked, who cares?

9   A recent variant on the traditional story of how cities arose, is the suggestion that the first city states were aggregations of gatherer hunters who congregated in river deltas where there were concentrations of seafood etc.[31].

10   Depending how transmissible is an infectious agent, it requires a specific size of human population before it can get established.

11   The other substantial relics of the middle ages in Europe are the cathedrals, most of which were built in a wave of competitive construction starting in about 1130 CE and lasting just over a century.

12   One exception is the 'Ulpian life-table' which consists of actuarial calculations used to determine annuities in the Roman Empire, and which have been used to suggest a life expectancy of 30 years.

13   I characterise debt as an evil here because it acts as a means of social control with its effects weighing most on the poor[22]. Financiers on the other hand may find debt quite desirable. It counts as assets on the balance sheet of a bank[33].

14   Some researchers have suggested on the basis of the recorded symptoms and dynamics of plague epidemics that they may have been caused by a viral haemorrhagic fever, related to Ebola[18] but this is generally disbelieved because *Yersinia pestis* DNA has been found in the skeletal remains of a number of the victims. However, based on the diversity of organisms that recurrently threaten to cause local epidemics or pandemics, it seems unlikely that all these epidemics were caused by the same pathogen.

15   This is the English name for a series of related conflicts referred to in Switzerland as the 'Schwabenkrieg'.

2. The Full Flush of Youth: Epidemics and Survival since the Enlightenment

"A good sewer.... a far nobler and a far holier thing... than the most admired Madonna ever painted." —John Ruskin

Most of the history described in Chapter 1, consisted of economic boom and bust cycles, and cycles of epidemics and plagues. These were often interlinked, with war or pestilence the cause of economic crashes, and no sign of escape from either treadmill. The first sign of an escape in terms of health may have been when the European aristocracy pulled away from the rest of society during the Enlightenment of the 18th century. Health effects of economic inequality in earlier periods are largely unknown, with patchy data from as far back as Ancient Rome [25], indicating that richer and higher-status people had somewhat better health in some periods but not others. However, not even the rich and powerful had long lives. In 16th and 17th century England the aristocracy had, if anything, worse survival than everyone else (Figure 1). Then, starting in the 18th century, at least in England a substantial difference in life-expectancy[1] opened between the aristocracy and the rest.

Figure 2 gives the whole time series of life-expectancy at birth for the UK since the start of the 19th century[2].

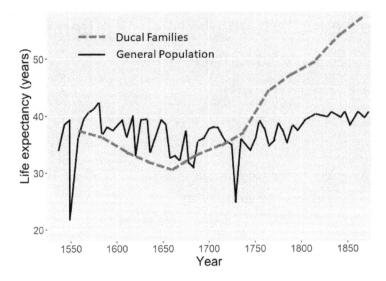

Figure 1. Life expectancy for the English population and for ducal families[3]

There were many large epidemics in the 19th century which continued to take many lives (Figure 2).[4] resulting in wiggles in the time-series of the UK life expectancy. There were also economic boom-bust cycles in industrialised countries[5]. Then, in the last few decades, the sanitation revolution saw a massive reduction in infectious disease, including the elimination of cholera and typhoid as public health problems.

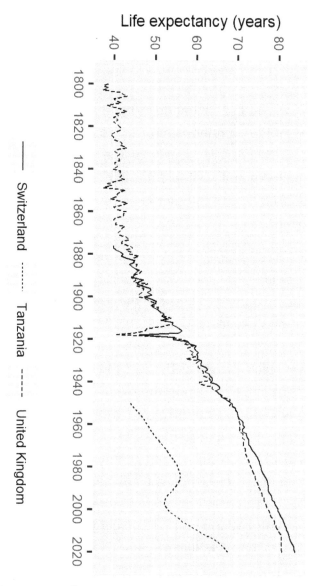

Figure 2. Life expectancy in the United Kingdom, Switzerland and Tanzania

The wiggles were smoothed out and there were tremendous improvements in life expectancy in industrialised countries that continued into the 21st century.

Deaton's book on the sanitation revolution is entitled '*The Great Escape*' [25], a reference to the escape from a WW2 prison camp that is the subject of the 1963 film of the same name[6]. But the escape from hunger and infectious disease associated with the sanitation revolution was of far greater significance.

Just as the great escape seemed to have taken off, In the second decade of the 20th century, every major industrialised country, including the UK, experienced a substantial crash in life expectancy. This was due to both World War I and the influenza pandemic that began while the war was still in progress. This was the last pandemic big enough to leave a clear dip in the trend in life-expectancy in Europe and North America. Even without the effect of the pandemic, life expectancy in the richest countries of the world in 1920 was still only comparable with that in the poorest and most AIDS-stricken nowadays. The smooth increase since then, in the case of the UK with just a smaller dip during World War II [25], and a flattening out in the last decade, is unparalleled in human history[7].

The trend in life expectancy for Switzerland (Figure 2). is like that for the UK, but without the dips due to the two world wars, which Switzerland avoided. By comparing the curves for the UK and Switzerland in the 1914-1919 period, it is possible to see that Spanish Influenza was comparable in its effect on life expectancy to the effect of the First World War in the UK. After 1960 Switzerland pulled ahead of the UK, with a noticeable further pulling away in the last decade.

The third line on Figure 2 shows life expectancy in Tanzania since 1950s (earlier data being unreliable, though there is evidence that the 1918 influenza hit hard there too) showing a typical African low-income country pattern. Initially, survival was like that in mid-19th century Europe, then during the last part of the colonial period, and the first decades of independence, there were parallel improvements to those in the industrialised world. Then the HIV epidemic, debt crises, and structural adjustment of the 1980s led to a prolonged dip in the curve, less deep than that in the second decade of the 20th century in the UK[8], but much more prolonged.

Since the 1990s there has been a steep increase in life-expectancy (and decrease in fertility) in Tanzania, as in most other low-income countries). This demographic transition mirrors that a century earlier in Europe, but deliberate health interventions are playing a much more direct role. HIV treatments were discovered and eventually used. Many of the infections that had been killing children were prevented by vaccination (measles, bacterial pneumonia) or were effectively treated with simple interventions (diarrhoeal disease treated with oral rehydration). Chapter 6 goes into the detail of part of this success story: insecticide-treated nets against malaria.

All this analysis has summarised the trends in health with the single statistic of life expectancy at birth[9]. This hides the change that was going on at the same time, in terms of which diseases were important. In high mortality settings it was mainly infectious disease in children, shifting to chronic disease like diabetes and heart disease in older people as life expectancy improved. There is no space here to go into the details of that, except to note that infectious disease has never gone away. Even before Covid-19 provided a forthright example, many of the infirm elderly in the industrialised world, were still dying with infections that they would have brushed off, had they not suffered from underlying chronic disease.

Globally, epidemics of infectious disease have never stopped. Smallpox was eliminated in Europe in 1953, but elsewhere epidemics continued until the last case in Somalia in 1977[42]. The late 20th century saw epidemics of malaria in countries that suspended indoor residual spraying programs, and recurrent meningitis epidemics across the Sahel zone of Africa. Elsewhere in the world, dengue outbreaks have been increasing in frequency, and geographical scope.

The difference between the period after the middle of the 20th century and that before, is that we have learnt how to avert some of them: smallpox was eradicated by a heroic vaccination effort[43]; at the time of writing, polio hangs on only in Afghanistan and Pakistan. Other diseases that caused epidemics in Europe in the past, including malaria, plague, typhoid, and cholera, still cause epidemics elsewhere, but can be relatively easily treated by chemotherapy so they do not cause epidemics in places with good health care systems. We have become rather good at isolating ourselves from environmental reservoirs of infection, but anyone who thinks that the decades since the eradication of smallpox represent a period free of major epidemics in the industrialised world, has

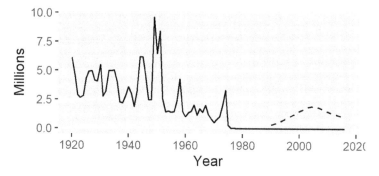

Figure 3. Annual deaths from major epidemic diseases during the last century (global

conveniently forgotten HIV[10] (Figure 3).

There has never been a period when new epidemic disease did not arise, but it is not surprising that during the Covid-19 pandemic there are prophets of the apocalypse claiming that this epidemic is a consequence of lifestyles that separate us from nature.

There have been many predictions that we would sooner or later face a catastrophic pandemic. Notably, Laurie Garrett's 1994 'The Coming Plague'[13], which summarised the history of epidemics in the second half of the 20th century. Garrett proposed that the health transition of the 1950s-60s in the industrialised world had led to an ecologically impoverished world in which humans had lost their immunity and made themselves vulnerable. A whole literature of outbreak novels has bought into this plotline. Since then, from this perspective, there have been various near misses (or hits, if you were unfortunate enough to be caught by avian influenza, SARS-1, MERS, Zika, or Ebola). But epidemics have never gone away in the meningitis belt of the Sahel, or the places where you can get Rift Valley fever, nor have any of the other encephalitis-causing viruses that flare up here and there across the world. Or in the (growing) area of the world vulnerable to dengue fever. The list goes on.

There may be places in the world where exposure to endemic coronaviruses provides protection against Covid-19. But it is a mistake to think that we would have been free of pandemics if we had remained in some idyllic state of nature. We can never know how many epidemics, with different ecology would have occurred if we had not industrialised, and a brief glance at Figure 2 should give pause for thought to any readers who are sceptical about progress. There will always be epidemics, but over time humans have grown better at dealing with them.

---

1   Much of this book uses life-expectancy as a summary of the state of health of a population. Broadly speaking, patterns of health measured in other ways (such as by disease rates, or the numbers of deaths of children) are likely to follow similar patterns. A brief explanation is found in Chapter 8 of what life expectancy is and is not, its limitations and the reasons why, if you need to summarise health with one number, this is probably the best one.

2   Figure 2 is based on free material from gapminder.org, CC-by license[36].

3   This plot was redrawn from [25], which in turn cited as sources Wrigley [37] for the estimates for the general population, and Hollingsworth [38] for the ducal families.

4   Historians long argued about whether the industrial revolution resulted in an improvement or deterioration of wellbeing (see for instance E.P. Thompson's 'The Making of the English Working Class'[39]), a question of intense contemporary relevance, since urbanisation means that about one in six of the global population are now living in urban slums[40], paralleling the 19th century urbanisation in the UK and parts of central Europe. This question has been answered empirically for the areas of early industrialisation in the UK, where the early stages of industrialisation between 1825-50 indeed reduced life expectancy but then there was a recovery[37]. This dip is not evident in the national level life expectancies shown in Figure 1 and Figure 2 presumably because industrial areas at first contributed only a small proportion of the population. Adult height, a measure of chronic malnutrition declined through most of the nineteenth century in industrialising countries[41].

5 Some European conservatives bundled left-wing revolutionaries, prostitution, and disease, all of which were associated with crisis, into the same mental category.

6   It is a great title. But of course, we have not completely escaped mortality, and after the real escape most of the escapees were recaptured and shot.

7   In comparison with earlier wars World War II was associated with fewer epidemics of infectious disease in Europe. In South East Asia and the Pacific epidemic malaria played possibly a decisive role in the war, striking soldiers from North America, Europe and Japan who had no immunity to the disease. Control of supplies of anti-malarial drugs was an important strategic issue.

8   The Spanish Influenza also struck Africa hard, as documented by horror stories about what happened in hospitals, but there are no reliable data with which to estimate its demographic impact.

9   See the explanation in Chapter 8 of why this text mainly discusses life expectancy and not how many people had different diseases.

10   The AIDS pandemic has killed 32 million people so far, with a demographic impact that dwarfs that of Covid-19, especially in Southern Africa. However, AIDS is a niche disease in industrialised countries, so has never required massive interventions across the whole population in Europe and North America.

3. The Importance of a Good Job (or of avoiding a bad one)

"Life is a dream for the wise, a game for the fool, a comedy for the rich, a tragedy for the poor. "—Sholem Aleichem

It is tempting to try to compare the health trends in the last two centuries that were described in Chapter 2, with economic indicators to see how they relate. This relationship is difficult to interpret. It is not obvious whether economic development drove health improvements, or *vice versa*, not least because of technological change. When new technologies are continually arising, what could have been done with a given amount of money at one time point is different from what can be done later, when the new possibilities are in place. Technological changes that underpinned the sanitation revolution of the late 19th century included flush toilets, vaccines, and disinfectants[1]. Some technologies, like sewage systems, were invented in the ancient world but were neglected in Europe for millennia.

There is an enormous literature showing that that poorer people in low- and middle-income countries have poorer health and poorer access to health care e.g. [45] on most indicators that have been analysed. It makes sense to believe that social change and health improvements depend on a small number of key technologies, and that in much of the world poverty restricts access to some these.

Medical innovations, especially antibiotics, are obviously important but non-medical technologies can also have big effects. Air-conditioners enable people in hot places to protect themselves from heat waves. More efficient heating and insulation protects us from the cold. Less obviously, but very likely at least as important, improved communications increase our capabilities [46] and technological innovations like the internet generally give us more control over our own lives (see below)[2]. For this reason, mobile phones may be a key contributor to improvements in health in low-income countries[3].

In contrast, by the 1970s it was widely supposed that big transformations in health in the rich world were a matter of history. Looking back over the previous century Thomas McKeown [47] pointed out that effective curative medicine, using innovations like antibiotics, largely arrived in the 20th century, after the big improvements in health resulting from preventative health interventions. He attributed much of the improvement to improved nutrition. In the UK this was used by the political left to challenge the special status of the medical elite and of curative medicine; social development with preventive health interventions, improvements in welfare and in education, especially of women (mothers' education correlates especially strongly with child health), was what was needed. Conversely, in the USA McKeown's findings were taken up by the libertarian right as an argument that economic growth (and by illogical extension liberalized markets, see Chapter 5) is all that is needed to improve health[4].

The rich world which mostly had universal health care coverage and had escaped from infectious disease, so some people wrongly assumed disparities in health by social class had ended. These were still pervasive, especially in the UK [48]. Material poverty preventing people accessing essential things did not explain this. Alternative explanations, that poorer people have an unhealthy culture, or that the causal relationship is in the direction that healthy people become rich, leaving the poor behind could also only explain a limited part of the effect[49].

Since the Black Report it has become apparent that much of the effect economic equality on health, results from anxiety and stress associated with insecurity and social status. The first findings (by Michael Marmot, Figure 4,[5, 50]),were that British civil servants [5] in more prestigious positions had much lower death rates than lower status civil servants, and that less educated Scandinavians have higher mortality than more educated ones (Figure 5,[51]), even if all the other obvious factors like age, smoking are allowed for.

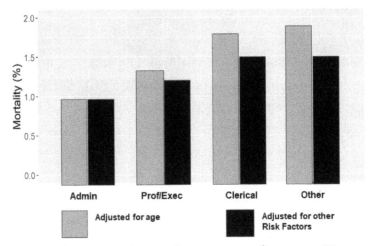

Figure 4. Coronary heart disease mortality over 25 years in the first Whitehall study showing contribution of risk factors to the social gradient.[6]

Further studies along the same lines, and thorough analysis of what could explain them[50], show that the effects on mortality arise because occupation and educational attainment affect social status which in turn affects levels of anxiety and the extent to which we experience a sense of control over our own lives[6].

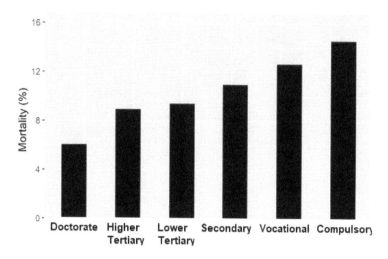

Figure 5. Mortality according to level of education in Swedish men 1991-6.[7]

These psychosocial factors are key risk factors for circulatory problems like high blood pressure and heart disease, which cause much of the mortality in high income countries. Debt is also a huge stress factor, that systematically blights the lives of those who have fallen into its clutches[52]. While the vast burden of disease assigned to mental health problems, does not lead to very many deaths coded with mental health diagnoses[53], it does shorten lives. The very direct effect on life expectancy of suicide (a connection already noted in the 19th century by Emile Durkheim[54]) is only one, relatively infrequent, way in which mental illness shortens lives.

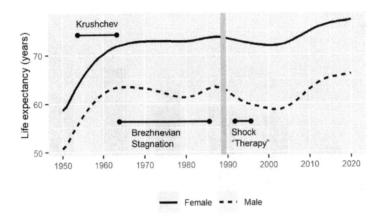

Figure 6. Life expectancy in Russia, 1950-2020.[8]

In contrast to contemporary situations of inequality, situations, where even the affluent have lived in an oppressive milieu, as in Brezhnev's Russia (1964-1982, Figure 6) (and presumably even more so under Stalin), or in Tudor England[9], there was little or no health benefit of being at the top of the heap, so life expectancy was depressed for everyone (Figure 1).

Conversely, early phases of consumerism, when substantial numbers of people have an enhanced range of choices (albeit over things that appear banal and unimportant to others who grew up in a consumer society), are associated with increases in average life-expectancy (e.g. Russia in the Khrushchev period, Figure 6). Lifespans have increased rapidly in East Asia with the growth of the middle class. When consumerism becomes established however, the frenzy of competitive acquisition feeds into the debt and status anxiety experienced by those at the bottom of the heap[5], thus increasing the burden of chronic disease and reinforcing the relationship of inequality with health.

Since the late 1970s the standard model of neoclassical economics gradually increased its power. By at the end of the Cold War, the conservative historian Francis Fukuyama could receive international plaudits for *"The end of history"*, an inverted pseudo-Marxist thesis that the capitalists had won, and that it was good[56]. We had reached the end of history, he wrote [10]. Fukuyama continues to be influential in the United States[11] even though the 9/11 attacks, and the subsequent wars in the Middle East had already made it obvious that this idea was ridiculous, but shrugging off the financial crisis of 2008, capitalism has continued to rule the world.

In politics, the mid-20th century can be seen as having been a prolonged conflict between more or less totalitarian theories of everything (Communism, Fascism, neoclassical economics)[57]. There was an interlude after World War II, 'Les Trente Glorieuses' when the ruling classes in the western world called a truce in the class war. Scandinavian countries then developed probably the most successful social models that the world has ever seen. Meanwhile the media in anglophone countries give the impression that they consider social democracy, Scandinavian style a second-rate variant of capitalism that burdened with unnecessary regulation [12]. This is despite the worse performance of deregulated societies on indicators that matter to people's well-being.

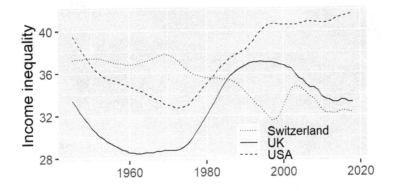

Figure 7. Income Inequality (as measured by the Gini index) over time[13]

Some financiers and politicians paused to think when Thomas Piketty's *'Capital in the Twenty-First Century'*[58] and then Branko Milanovic' *'Global Inequality'*[59] became best-sellers, documenting in impressive detail the trend since the 1960s in the distribution of income and wealth in the industrialised world, especially in the Anglophone countries, in favour of the wealthiest (Figure 7)[14]. This contrasts with the previous century when inequality had tended to lessen.

Milanovic documented how globally, the incomes of the people in the middle of the distribution especially the burgeoning middle class of China and India, grew massively in the period since 1990 (Figure 8).

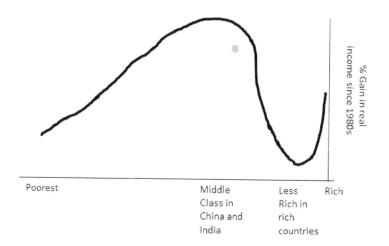

Poorest   Middle   Less   Rich
                  Class in   Rich in
                  China and   rich
                  India   countries

Figure 8. Schematic of Milanovic' Elephant Diagram: the pattern of gain in income by position within the global income distribution, late 1980s-2010.[15]

So, while the 99% in the rich countries may largely perceive a slow erosion of incomes and of economic prospects, this is not the experience of most of the rest of the world's population. Nevertheless, a small minority of people have captured most of the wealth increase, and the continuing improvements in average life expectancy in industrialised countries are therefore not because people have more money[16]. Most of them do not

Few of the readers of Piketty and Milanovic' books seem to have thought about the fact that this inequality was killing people in their hundreds of thousands.

The evidence for this comes partly from geographical comparisons of measures of health with income inequality as measured here by the Gini index. Figure 9 is a comparison of national level statistics for the Organisation for Economic Co-operation and Development (OECD, i.e. wealthy) countries. There is a downward trend in life-expectancy and an upward trend in infant mortality with increased inequality, though something else is obviously of importance in some of the low survival countries.

In both plots the four countries with the highest levels of inequality (Turkey, USA, Chile, and Lithuania) stand out as having adverse health outcomes. Comparisons of US states show similar patterns demonstrating that this is not an artefact of how the world is divided up into pieces [50].

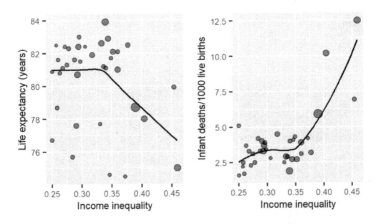

Figure 9. National life expectancy and infant mortality rates by income inequality (Gini index, OECD countries).[17]

To summarise this important and substantial literature in four sentences: stress and anxiety are major determinants of health status, independent of material well-being in terms of nutrition, health-oriented behaviour or environmental exposures. This leads to poorer health among those with less money, wherever wealth provides more control over your own life, and especially where the impoverished are marginalised and stressed. Particularly relevant cases are contemporary Anglophone countries where the growing precariat depends on casual work and the gig economy. The poor die sooner and it is not their own   fault.

1   Germ theory propagated by Louis Pasteur in France and Robert Koch in Germany provided the rationale for why these interventions work, but this was not a simple case of basic theory informing applied science, which in turn informed practice. Rather, the theory followed behind much of the practice. Pasteur's key work on human diseases began with his work on anthrax in the 1870s, while Koch was active from the 1880s onwards, but the clean-up began in the mid-19th century after panics about unclean environments, with imaginary connections often drawn between prostitution, left-wing agitation, smells, and disease. The seminal example of how the English physician John Snow identified contaminated water as the cause of the 1854 cholera epidemic in London, shows that public health interventions can be effective even when the biology is not understood. The cholera bacillus, Vibrio cholerae was first isolated in the same year[44], but these findings were first widely disseminated by Koch, 30 years later. Florence Nightingale, the social reformer and pioneer statistician remembered as a folk-heroine in the UK for her clean-up of military hospitals in the Crimean War, continued to believe in the miasma theory of disease transmission.

2   Although they can also be stressors and sources of inequity, especially for people who are struggling with new technology, or are trapped in the gig economy.

3   Mobile phones have had transformative effects in for poor people, not just because they can be used to disseminate messages, but because they enable people to be included in many ways, for instance learning about opportunities and about the market prices of what they produce.

4   McKeown's claim that curative medicine is of secondary importance for health transitions, does not argue for marketisation like that in the USA where curative medicine has grown the most.

5   A group among whom material deprivation is very unlikely to be important. They could all afford to satisfy their basic needs.

6   Redrawn from [5]. Mortality rates are relative to those of administrators. The grey bars are estimates allowing for age differences, the black bars additionally allow for differences in smoking, systolic blood pressure, plasma cholesterol, height, and blood sugar. The residual gradient after allowing for all these risk factors is attributable to the psychosocial effects of occupational status[5, 50].

7   Percentage of men aged sixty-four in 1990 who died up to December 1996, by level of education[51], redrawn from [5].

8   The grey vertical line corresponds to the end of the Soviet Union. Based on free material from gapminder.org, CC-by license[36].

9   Wolf Hall[55], Hilary Mantel's fictionalisation of the experience of the Tudor aristocracy is widely thought to have captured the mood of a period in English history when any personal autonomy was overshadowed by the oppressive fear of hell if they jumped the wrong way in the religious conflicts of the time, or of being burnt at the stake if they didn't. A single error in Tudor power politics often meant execution.

10   I am relying on reviews and Wikipedia to infer the content of this book. I never bought it.

11   Illustrating the fact that the Trump regime is not breaking new ground in placing dangerous fantasists close to power.

12   The extent to which this lie has taken hold demonstrates that fake news in politics is not some invention of the Trump era. It should be one of the great scandals of our time that this idea has been consistently propagated by supposedly responsible media like the Economist, CNN, or the BBC.

13   Based on free material from gapminder.org, CC-by license[36].

14   Figure 7 extends the plot for patterns of inequality in the UK and the USA up to 2018 and includes the line for Switzerland. The inexorable increase in inequality has continued in the USA up to the present. The pattern for the UK shows that changes of government can make a difference, and the Swiss time-series confirms that increases in inequality during peacetime are by no means inevitable.

15   Schematic based on the diagram in[59].

16   The improvements in health are mainly the result of the transformative technologies that continue to increase human potential, but most of the scientists who develop these are not among the financial beneficiaries. Some scientists form start-up companies, which generally increases stress, without necessarily providing financial rewards.

17   Data from OECD [60]

4. The Roles of Natural Science and Fiction

"You might think that this ..... outcome would cause much anguished soul-searching among economists, as a basic assumption of their theory had been successfully challenged. But this is not the way things work in social science, including both psychology and economics." — Daniel Kahneman[61]

I just awoke from a vivid dream set in a lockdown, where people connected with each other via the internet to form a utopian community, in which they exchanged without money and there was no hierarchy, just gifts sent back and forth electronically. The gifts were stories the people had written, artwork they created, jokes they told each other, or photographs they took of the natural world they found flourishing around themselves. Some of the people in the community were also still performing essential work, producing or distributing food, in the old style economy, but they didn't need to consume so very much of these products, so it was not a big problem that some of them were unable or unwilling to contribute. Maybe they organised rotas so that everyone who wanted could work in the vegetable fields now and again or drive a distribution van.

In the dream, there was no evidence of a pandemic, no dead, nor dying, and the members of the utopian community were blissfully unaware of the other people, who because of one misfortune or another were excluded, either because they had no internet connection, or could not adjust to the demands of a world that lived in cyberspace. The members of the community did not watch the television news, so they had no idea of any of this. Most of all, they had no idea that the economy had tanked. If someone had told them that the economy had tanked, they would have responded with a puzzled, "So what?".

In the dream, the lockdown came to an end, and the government told anyone who mentioned it that the utopian community had never existed. Since everything the community had produced and shared was virtual, it was hard to argue with this (the date-stamp on virtual artefacts produced during the lockdown might have been faked), so most people believed the myth that it never happened, and returned to the lives they had led before.[1]

In the real world as in the dream, there are some things that are studied by the natural sciences and could be detected by a Martian with the correct measuring devices. There are other things that the visitor from another planet would not know were there. The historian Yuval Noah Harari contends that all large-scale human cooperation systems including religions, political structures, and legal institutions that exist because of people come into this category and can be classified as fiction[9][2].

In the natural sciences, if we build a mathematical model of a phenomenon, we start by assembling data about it, either by experiment, or by observing what is going on. For instance, when we assembled a micro-simulation model of malaria[62] we pulled together all the quantitative information we could easily find from field studies measuring each transition in the life cycle of the parasite, and tried to make all the relationships in our computer model match this data as closely as possible[63]. With some parts of the model it was difficult to understand the patterns in the data. For instance, however many mosquitoes are biting people, it is extremely unusual for every single person in a field study to get infected with malaria. So as epidemiologists, we used a statistical model that simply reproduced the relationship between these variables found in the data [64]. That is the sort of thing that would make chemists or physicists uncomfortable, because it means that we do not really understand in biological terms what is going on. It made me uncomfortable too, so I embarked on a series of different analyses[64, 65] (please excuse the self-citations) to try to work out what the explanation might be, before realising that this was an inevitable result of the fact that some people are bitten by mosquitoes far more often than others[66], and that a model including chance variation that explicitly captures this[67, 68] is theoretically the best way to go.

Econometric modelling sometimes does the opposite, it starts with the theory, makes some predictions, then looks around for data to see if the real world obeys the theory. This amounts to operating in Harari's realm of fiction.

Mainstream neoclassical economics is a body of theory about how to allocate tradable resources among alternative ends largely built on assumptions of how humans behave in markets. The ideal economic man, is an agent who makes individual self-interested choices, based on perfect knowledge of the relevant alternatives. His choices are intended to maximize a personal utility function, which can easily end up being expressed in terms of money.

The Italian economist Vilfrido Pareto is credited with the insight that if the world were inhabited with these beings trading in unconstrained markets then none of them would be able to better their condition without making one of the others worse off. This ideal state is called Pareto optimality. But the world is not inhabited by such *homunculi*[3]. So why does Pareto's insight matter?

It matters because from these three assumptions, neoclassical economists have built a dogma that has taken over the world. As an example, I remember a presentation given about the introduction of competitive health insurance in the Netherlands, given at a health economics workshop in an Alpine ski resort[4]. The presentation began with a mathematical model of how economic man would behave in this situation. It was rather technical, and some people in the room switched off at that stage (presumably because they were tired after being on the slopes earlier in the day). The middle part of the presentation described what really happened in the Netherlands. The theory said that the Dutch should have spent their evenings tracking health insurance prices and switching from one provider to another[5]. That did not happen. On the other hand, the theory had provided an ideological cover for marketisation within the health sector, allowing private actors to cream off rents disguised as legitimate transaction costs. The conclusion of the presentation amounted to an inditement of the Dutch population for failing to properly optimise their personal utilities.

When I first learnt of utilitarianism as a teenager in the industrial West Yorkshire, it had seemed very much like common-sense. Around me was a world of regular employment in manufacturing industry that superficially corresponded to the imaginings of the 19th century philosophers Jeremy Bentham, John Stuart Mill, and their contemporaries who invented the calculus of utilities. The alternative 19th century model of Marx and Engels, which saw capitalism as the arena of class conflict, not utility maximisation, also seemed to make a lot of sense. This should not be a surprise, given that cities of the north of England provided much of their data [70], in particular the idea that exchange value arises from the labour that goes into production, (originating with another UK-based economist, Ricardo), but that workers are exploited by being paid much less[6], seemed a more promising starting point for understanding the economy. It had not been obvious then that the birthplaces of the industrial revolution were about to deindustrialise or that a version of the standard economic model that ignored all the inconvenient (for the rich) aspects of reality, was about to dominate political and economic discourse. Three decades later, in the Bernese Alps, it seemed obvious that any connection between labour, merit (whatever that is), and who gets to go to the top winter-sports resort[7], is strictly in the realm of imagination.

At the same meeting, I gave a rather pedestrian talk about some cost-effectiveness (see Chapter 6) calculations for malaria vaccines[71, 72][8]. Afterwards I shared a train compartment with some of the senior econometricians who had been present. They were curious about the incentives driving the funding of malaria programs, insisting that whoever was paying must be expecting an economic return. I tried to convince them that this could not be the case. How could utility-maximisation explain the eclectic distribution of contributions between different donors (for example Scandinavian governments with minimal economic interests in sub-Saharan Africa, and philanthropists)?[9]

We all changed trains (in Interlaken and Spiez), and I pondered over our completely different understandings of the role of modelling in guiding health programs. Natural science is a set of methodologies that allow for continual modification and updating of theories, in principle nothing is set in stone, and everything needs to be tested against evidence. In our work we tried to avoid making calls requiring value of life calculations (Chapter 7), except for simply assuming that it is better if fewer people die. It was not our job to decide whether a particular cost-effectiveness ratio (see Chapter 6) should translate into a decision to spend money on a vaccine[10]. But these econometricians seemed to think they should be planning whole health systems even though they have minimal understanding of how people behave or what really matters to them.

---

1   In case there seems to be something vaguely familiar about this dream, I should point out that there are some parallels with the plot of H.G. Wells 'The Time Machine', published in 1895.

2   I suspect Harari's[9] claim is an oversimplification but this is a pragmatic way to avoid going over centuries of philosophical debate about mind-body dualism and relativism.

3   Going through the characteristics of *economic man*, one by one, we find that his behaviour is in all respects unlike that of any human on our planet with the findings of behavioural economics[61, 69] providing the killing blow . In this version of the story I am allowing the homunculus to struggle through a further four chapters in order to outline some details of his pathology.

4   International meetings held in the Alps should in any case raise suspicions. They are an obvious case of market failure. Technical efficiency is reduced by the difficulties experienced by participants in concentrating at high altitude, especially after a day's skiing, and there are opportunity costs associated with the more complicated travel arrangements compared with meetings in urban areas (or in cyberspace).

5   The Dutch have had a reputation as avid traders since the Golden Age (I apologise for use of this term, which is currently being challenged in the Netherlands because the period was associated with slave trading). So, a system that anticipated people changing their health insurance to get a better deal should work in the Netherlands, if it would work anywhere. However, the Dutch people I know like to go out to bars in the evenings. Even the Dutch prefer life to Pareto optimality, if forced to make the choice (technically this could be addressed in the model by considering the opportunity cost of trading, but should the people who have better things to do with their lives get a worse deal than obsessive geeks?).

6   The labour theory of value didn't stand the test of time and as a born and bred Yorkshireman I have always found it hard to take seriously the idea that the working class of northern England had much potential for leading a socialist revolution. The results of the 2019 UK general election are consistent with the idea that some elements of political culture last a long time. Marx already understood that the English working class had far less propensity to revolution than workers elsewhere in Europe but it is probably a long time since Jeremy Corbyn read Marx.

7   We were about 150 km west of Davos, where the annual World Economic Forum is held.

8   Both the one malaria vaccine that is currently being deployed in pilot programmes [73] and various hypothetical vaccines with different biological effects.

9   I wanted to convince them that the rural poor of Africa do not even belong to Marx' reservoir of the unemployed, but I realised that mentioning Marx would have raised a red flag.

10 Conveniently, calculations of the effects of malaria interventions, measuring health in different ways (deaths, life-years lost, or DALYs), generally line-up[10].

5. The Cancer of Growthism in the Health Agenda

"Annual income twenty pounds, annual expenditure nineteen [pounds] nineteen [shillings] and six [pence], result happiness. Annual income twenty pounds, annual expenditure twenty pounds ought and six, result misery." — Charles Dickens [74]

When I began to work in the field of international health, in the late 1980s as a statistician in Papua New Guinea, it appeared to me, naïve newbie as I was, that a major, if not the main problem of rural development was that there was hardly any money in rural areas. It was still taken for granted in the rich world that the unemployed should receive enough money to live on, but just giving money to the poor was taboo in low income countries[1] (this seemed to reflect some unmentionable double standard).

Since giveaways were obviously out of the question, the obvious way to inject money into rural communities was to increase the pay of the teachers and primary health care staff. Almost all low-income countries face severe problems in retaining trained health staff and teachers in rural areas, because the pay is abysmal and sometimes does not even arrive, and rural areas are often unpleasant places to live. Almost everyone prefers to be in the capital, or a migrant worker in the industrialised world.

There were plenty of Non-Governmental Organisations (NGOs) and development agencies around on the look-out for projects so I wondered if some of them were supporting the local teachers and health centre workers, who would clearly be doing something useful if they had not been demoralised and diverted into corruption by the need to feed their families. Instead though a large part of what purported to be development, consisted of feeding the corruption and cutting off services to the poor, by introducing school fees into primary education and user fees into the health system.

Normally the performance of the economy is assessed via growth in GDP and anticipates progress in the shape of continually increasing economic activity. We are bombarded with statistics, generally not on the size of the economy (which would seem large), but on its rate of growth. Since it is assumed that technologies will make productivity increase, the economy needs to grow if levels of activity are not to decrease[2]. Sometimes however some people think it needs to shrink in order to grow.

In the late 1980s structural adjustment programs were in full swing. Just as in Southern Europe twenty years later, the governments of low-income countries had borrowed more money than they could afford to pay back[3], and the condition for cancelling the debts was to trash the public services. After a couple of decades, when enough statistics had been collected to demonstrate that structural adjustment programs generally do not work on their own terms[4], I was puzzled. I do not understand macro-economics, but I do understand basic statistics.

In a system with randomness, if it is perturbed it will tend to return towards the long-term average because of the phenomenon of regression towards the mean[5]. To take an extreme example: consider a patch of land with a tall building on. If you knock it down, the level is zero. There is nowhere else to go but up, so if anything happens at all, there will be growth. So even if the deterministic models used to justify the structural adjustment bear little relationship to a reality perfused with randomness, structural adjustment should have led to growth.

But it takes a very long time for an economy to get back to where it started from if it is knocked down. I illustrate this using data on GDP from Bolivia (Figure 10), where there was a complex economic crisis in the early 1980s[6]. The horizontal grey line in the top plot highlights that it took until 2005 for the Bolivian GDP to catch up to where it was in 1977 despite a pattern of growth rates over the period that at first sight just look like a lot of noise and aren't so different from those of Switzerland (bottom panel).

Growth in GDP is just not such a good indicator of what was going on. Indeed, in 1977 there was a steep negative growth in Switzerland (Figure 10) but it didn't have strange and perverse effects like those when the economy bottomed-out in Bolivia in the mid-1980s[7]. All kinds of bizarre things can happen when the economy of a poor country crashes.

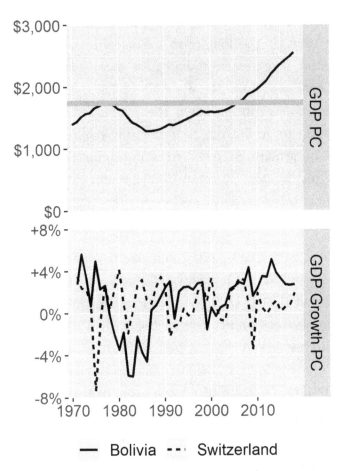

Figure 10. GDP and growth in GDP in Bolivia.[8]

Moving to Switzerland in 1991, I became interested in comparisons between Switzerland and the UK, the country where I was born. Over most of the last 30 years, GDP growth has been higher in the UK than in Switzerland (Figure 11), but on visiting the UK I have the impression that the infrastructure there has degraded or stood still, while that of Switzerland has massively improved. If anything, the salary differential, at least for scientists, has increased. This is because the UK has a boom and bust economy and Switzerland a counter-cyclical one where there is less variation over time in the growth rate (except for that dip in 1977). The absolute difference in GDP between Switzerland and the UK has increased.

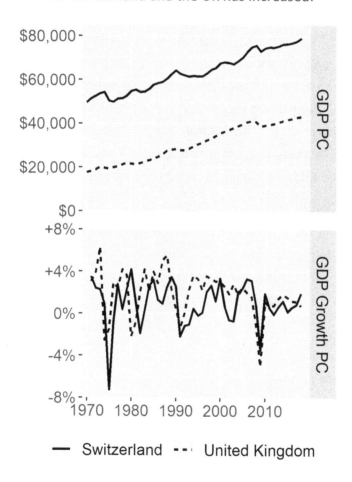

Figure 11. GDP and GDP growth: Switzerland and UK.[9]

Econometricians include some very smart mathematicians (after all this is the community that invented the Black-

Scholes equation)[10]. So, it is difficult to believe that they do not understand basic concepts like regression to the mean. But if you are fixated on growth, which is the rate of change of the thing you are really interested in[11], then it is easy to see how you might be confused about what is going on here. In fact, the really striking comparison to be extracted from Figure 10 and Figure 11 is the comparison of the trend in per capita GDP in Bolivia with that in Switzerland. In a plot with them both on the same linear scale, the time-series for Bolivia simply runs along at the bottom close to the horizontal. The annual increment in economic activity corresponding to a 4% growth rate in Bolivia, would barely register as a bump on the time series of GDP for Switzerland.

But why all this discussion of GDP, when most of us know that we live on a finite planet and believe that economic growth cannot continue indefinitely[12]? Isn't that all that needs to be said about it? And what has this to do with health?

Well, GDP happens to be quite a good predictor of life expectancy at country level, at least in comparison of poor countries with rich ones[13](Figure 12). This relationship is referred to as the Preston curve. The relationship is concave. Among countries with GDP above about $20,000 per annum, GDP is not very strongly related to life-expectancy. If the average wealth and income increase in poor countries, health will generally improve (unless the increase is all grabbed by a small minority), but if basic needs are already satisfied then more money is less important. So, we should be concerned that the GDP in Bolivia is so low. GDP in the rich world (and even more so, growth in GDP), the subject of so much political and media angst, especially in Anglophone counties, is hardly related to health and well-being at all. At the individual level, the message should be that if you have more than you need you are rich and should not be stressing about becoming richer. If you have less, then you have a serious problem.

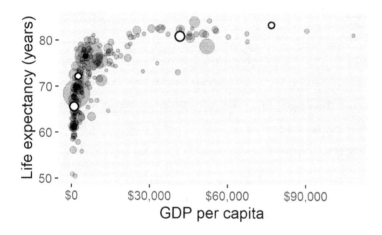

Figure 12. Life expectancy by country GDP[14]

Similarly, the enormous number of studies showing that poor people have poorer health (Chapter 3), make it obvious that relieving poverty will improve health, but the things that improve health are often not the same as those that provide an immediate stimulus to economic growth, and overall increases in wealth do not automatically reach the poorest. Spending money on the technology and infrastructure that underpinned the sanitation revolution, briefly described in Chapter 2, or the equivalent spending on research today, is accounted as input, rather than economic output[41], so they don't count as a particularly 'good thing' if progress is being assessed by GDP. These things pay off in health over a relatively short period, (though the health benefits continue to have benefits for a long time, as with 19th century water and drainage systems that continue to function).

Because of the relationship shown in Figure 12 the promotion of growth in low income countries often appears on the progressive side of the political spectrum; for many politicians, the alternative to assigning monetary values to welfare considerations is to let the market decide. The market may decide that people's health is essentially worthless, especially if the people concerned do not have any money or prospects of paid employment.

The public health community is used to being considered rather marginal, so it seemed like a step in the right direction when health is valued as something that might feed into the economy. The 1993 World Development Report[85], entitled 'Investment in Health' was consequently greeted with enthusiasm by many of those concerned about international health. It finally put health on the development agenda, along with finance, energy, agriculture, and the environment. The World Bank was finally taking health seriously, after more than a decade in which health programs had been among the main victims of structural adjustment programs.

We should not have needed the World Bank to tell us health is important. All these other sectors deal almost exclusively with things that are valued instrumentally, as means of achieving something else. It is a sign of the topsy-turvy thinking of international organizations, that among all these areas that we only value as means, the one that we value intrinsically should be struggling to get recognition.

Discussion of investment in health is now a commonplace in the international health community, but we rarely analyse what this means. The word 'investment' belongs to the vocabulary of economics, so on an ideological level perhaps this merely reflects the status that money-making has achieved as a pre-eminent activity, so 'investment' is one of those organisation-speak terms like 'business case', that are loosely applied and hence gradually lose their original meanings. To talk about an investment, though, implies that someone is expecting a return, probably a financial one. This should raise suspicions. By investing now, we will reap greater rewards at some time in the future. It is easy to see how this can apply to health and the concept appeals to progressives because it provides a rationale for preventive interventions, for instance vaccination. Vaccinating now provides a return later in terms of infections and illness averted. There is plenty of evidence that improving people's health improves their economic productivity, but the more this is examined in a disaggregated way, the clearer it is that this is not how anyone allocates resources for health, at least not in any country with pretentions to be civilized, other than the USA. It is abhorrent to even think that it might be. We do not size up whether the patient will perk up and overdeliver, when deciding whether to mend a broken leg.

When Jeffery Sachs initially promoted the mass distribution of free insecticide treated nets (ITNs, Chapter 6), an important part of his argument was that malaria has a massive effect on GDP growth. It had been clear for a very long time, that economic activity in the tropics is hindered by endemic disease. Gallup and Sachs[86] quantified this by comparing national level economic growth rates with data on how much malaria there is in each country and suggesting that eliminating malaria, would on average lead to a 3% increase in economic growth[15]. However, the inference that eliminating malaria will pay for itself, struggles with the fact that the health improvements are in different people in different places from those who become richer. At the same as advocating for eliminating malaria, which would primarily provide benefits to the people of rural Africa[10], Sachs was promoting a development model that sees connection with the rest of the world as the future for African economies. The boom would be (and has been) in tourist destinations, commercial agriculture, and port cities like Dar-es-Salaam[88] (which always had a much lower malaria incidence than the rural hinterland[89]).

It is just as well that this thinking was not joined-up. A consistent and informed advocate of the human capital approach would presumably analyse which people should receive the investment in order to maximise productivity. The wretched of the earth, whose needs are surely the greatest, and whose health issues can most cheaply be addressed[16], would have been ignored because they are not very well connected to the global economy, except for being perceived as a reservoir of infectious disease. We are not all equal in terms of our potential economic contributions, sometimes because of systematic disadvantage, such as racism or sexism, sometimes because of chance (where we are), so the concept of human capital is fundamentally inegalitarian[17].

Investment is about creating debts. Typically, the investee takes out a loan from a bank, which sooner or later is meant to be repaid. The debtor is obliged to work to repay the loan. When the investment is in the form of money paid into government programs, but the return is in health it is not so obvious how this is meant to happen, especially if the people whose health will benefit are hardly likely to become large-scale consumers or pay income tax. Unlike poll-tax systems which operate to indebt individuals[18] it seems like the debt is meant to lock whole countries into debt bondage. Underlying this is the logic of globalisation, an insatiable process of incorporating ever more of the world's people into a unitary system of exploitation. Except that the neoclassical economists see this as a benevolent process, with ever more people being enabled to participate in a system that brings Pareto optimality (Chapter 4) ever closer.

Where there is a donation, rather than a loan, it seems strange to use the language of 'investment'. For instance, the following statement from the Bill and Melinda Gates Foundation from October 2018 looks at first sight like an innocent endorsement of the value of human life (but read the endnotes):

"Human capital is an important component of economic growth. Investments in human capital add up to large benefits for economies—countries become richer[19] as more human capital accumulates[20]. Human capital is an important input to technological innovation and long-run growth. ..... investment on the health and education of girls is key......not educating girls costs countries $15 to $30 trillion in lifetime productivity and earnings."

Similarly, the conclusion from 1993 World Development Report[90]:

"Governments need to foster an economic environment that enables households to improve their own health."

But then we read that there should be:

"More diversity and competition in the financing and delivery of health services"

This should be controversial to say the least when the evidence is examined on which health systems perform the best. There is much debate about health care finance. Especially in those countries with overwhelming debt crises, combined with state-funded national health services, there is intense lobbying to find ways of reducing costs, linked to pressure to open the health sector in one way or another to private markets. In industrialised countries state-funded national health services represent the cheapest approach to financing health care[21]. Market approaches in the health sector are well known to be distorted by pervasive and unavoidable uncertainties, asymmetric information, all kinds of externalities and the special role of physicians[22]. There will always be ways to make health care more efficient (like those pursued by the UK's National Institute for Health and Clinical Excellence, NICE) but alternative financing approaches will generally increase expenditure on health care. They will generally also increase the potential for private profit. Some (most?) of the pressure for privatisation is in bad faith.

We are constantly bombarded with the message that *'Capital is Good'*. I remember as a child being puzzled by the daily TV news reports on house prices and stock-markets. It was always reported as a good thing when there is a bull market, and when house prices increase, even though it is obvious that a price increase is always a downside for the buyer. The bull market increases inequality and places a greater proportion of resources and political power in the control of a selfish minority. When house prices increase, many people are disadvantaged. Especially those who would like to own real estate but are not able to buy.

There again, much of what believes itself to be capitalist is not. In low income countries, much of the health budget comes from international development assistance[23] and philanthropy (especially the Bill & Melinda Gates Foundation). This forms only a small proportion of development assistance, but a large part of health expenditure in low income countries.

Much of the world's economy is now part of the philanthropic sector, and the rules by which this operates are not the same as those of either a socialist or a market logic. Philanthropy has much in common with development assistance, and indeed philanthropic foundations often work together with both multilateral and bilateral governmental development agencies, but there is no escaping from the role of chance events in the outcomes of philanthropy. There are a very small number of extremely rich individuals, which means that it matters how many of them (like Bill and Melinda Gates, or Warren Buffet) realise that becoming the richest individuals in the world doesn't provide immortality, and aspire to translate their wealth into benefits for the rest of humanity. Others decide to translate it into bizarre vanity projects like sending space flights to Mars; or, like the Koch brothers, into promoting insidious ideologies. The latter category continues to intensify its exploitative business models even when this provides them personally with no incremental benefit in terms of anything that is worth having.

Philanthropy represents a problem for neoclassical economists. The marginal utility of additional money is low for people who are extremely rich, so giving a larger proportion away makes more sense if you are rich[24]. But it is quite impossible to explain how billionaires spend their money within models of utility maximisation[94] because there is a huge role of chance. There are only a few billionaires, with a highly skewed distribution of wealth among them. What one billionaire thinks is rational for them to do, another may consider nuts, and *vice versa*, and these personal whims dramatically affect the lives of billions of people. The composition of the overall portfolio of philanthropic projects therefore depends a lot on chance. One personality trait that is probably essential if you want to become extremely rich, is a large dose of self-confidence, so each individual billionaire is likely to overestimate how smart they are relative to everyone else, and to underestimate the role of random events in how they acquired their wealth. This leads to a tendency to overestimate how much it is possible to control things, and to underestimate the roles of chance. Biographers retrospectively write surveys of the careers of the extreme rich, identifying the key decisions that worked out and writing them into self-help books. But vast numbers of other people might have made similar decisions or followed the advice in the self-help books and gone nowhere or ended up on the street. The extreme rich thus also overestimate the extent to which philanthropy can achieve extraordinary goals[25]. If many millions of people aspire to become billionaires, then some of them will make it. If a single billionaire aspires to achieve the extremely chancy objective of sending humans to Mars, the chances of success are negligible[26].

Maybe the growthist agenda in health is just a phase that will go away, and the buy-in to it from foundations like Gates' is an oversight. Ideologies in development change more over time than they do in space, despite the conclusion of Hirschman, one of the doyens of post-WW2 development, that what works varies enormously from one place to another[96]. It might seem obvious that this should be the case because the global South has had less exposure to the homogenizing effect of globalisation. In the absence of lockdowns, it is much harder to travel internationally within Africa than within Europe. Although Africa may appear rather uniform to Europeans[27], these places are very different from one another. Instead of embracing this diversity though, those of us from northern countries who spend part of our lives in the South are expected to return to the countries we came from, where we become global development experts, believing that what we learnt in one place has universal validity. Europeans would find it bizarre if an African 'European Studies' expert, who had spent a couple of years in Ireland, was advising the Bulgarians on what to do about Covid-19. Rather than setting global goals and targets like growth rates, the need is to concentrate on what works in terms of achieving meaningful health and development in each different place.

When we are hired to model cost-effectiveness by the philanthropy/development assistance world (Chapter 5), we are usually asked to provide results from societal perspective (if there is any recognition that the perspective matters), and what is possibly appreciated by most of us (including Bill Gates) is that the main value of wealth, is to achieve health. What value would money have for a moribund billionaire dying of an incurable disease? From this perspective the health even of the most wretched of the earth is to be valued as an end. Accumulation of assets by those whose needs are already satisfied, is a means. But to what end?

---

1   Three decades later, giving money to the poor became a fashionable development strategy which seems to be working in many places[75].

2   The assumption that economic activity is what matters means that policy is framed as a set of choices between growth and the scrap heap of unemployment. Alternatives to endless increase in production, like wholesale shifts of society away from traditional employment models (for instance, as suggested by Jeremy Rifkin[76]) are not even considered.

3   The organisation of international finance and the institutionalised greed of the finance sector are responsible for debt crises. Essentially governments of low-income countries can only borrow money if they offer high interest rates. When they do so banks pour in loans because of the high rate of return, even though there would appear to be a high risk of default. When the default happens, the creditors hold all the cards and frequently get bailed out. Because there is a good chance of a bailout, they pour in crazy amounts of money into the next round of lending because they believe they will be bailed out again and are taking no risks. There is a lot of literature on this.

4   Effects of structural adjustments on life expectancy appear as characteristic dips in plots of life expectancy over time (see Figure 2 for Tanzania though this was compounded by HIV, and Figure 6 for Russia). It is sobering to consider how large an infectious disease epidemic needs to be to achieve a comparable effect. The 'Shock Therapy' strategy is associated with Jeffrey Sachs[77]; in the Russian case it may or may not have succeeded in curing the economy, but either way many of the patients died.

5   In any time-series where the values depend on chance, extreme outcomes tend to be followed by more moderate ones.

6   I use the Bolivian crisis to illustrate the comparison between the use of GDP growth as an indicator and GDP itself. This crisis was not a typical debt crisis. It had multiple causes with the main symptom being hyperinflation. Jeffrey Sachs was the main adviser to the Bolivian government involved in the eventual stabilisation[78].

7   I also selected the Bolivian example because I experienced some of the bizarre fallout myself. A fictionalised excerpt from my Bolivian diary appeared as a short-story in 2011[79].

8   Data from World Bank[80].

9   Data from World Bank[80].

10   The Black-Scholes model is a mathematical model for financial markets used for pricing derivative investments[81]. The use of it is thought to have been a major contributor to the 2008 crash[33]. The traders had forgotten (or not received) warnings about the behaviour of non-linear models in unusual parts of the parameter space. I understand why they have not apologised. I am only now coming clean about fitting a dodgy non-linear model for the behaviour of a dust sampling device in my first job as a young statistician[82]. Maybe some of the exposure values in environmental epidemiology studies are inaccurate because of my bravado. Sorry.

11   For the moment, we ignore the reality that the size of the economy should in any case not be anybody's target.

12   The argument that finite physical resources impose a limit on economic growth, first popularised by the Club of Rome in 1972 [83] still has a lot of traction. However, if sustainable electricity sources can be harnessed, it is not so obvious what is the limit to growth in cyberspace, or what are the health implications. Much internet activity is via social media which people don't pay for, very likely increasing the disconnect between economic activity and well-being[84].

13   Among countries with high GDP, GDP itself is no longer a good predictor of life expectancy. Inequality then matters much more (Chapter 3, [6])

14   The bubbles are proportional to the size of the population, the highlighted points correspond to the four countries of Tanzania, Bolivia, UK, and Switzerland. Based on free material from gapminder.org, CC-by license[36].

15   This paper uses a simple application of regression analysis, that cannot test the alternative explanation that correlation of malaria with GDP growth is because it is reduced by urbanisation and improved housing. More recently models that can infer the direction of causality have also been applied to this problem[87]. These broadly support Gallup and Sachs'[86] estimate of the effect of malaria on GDP growth.

16   Where people have almost no access to services, even provision of a low-cost minimal improvement can make considerable difference. The 1993 World Development Report [90] advocated targeting expenditure at the most cost-effective interventions e.g. infectious disease and malnutrition. This makes sense, but the stated ultimate objective was to improve the economy not health. Mission statements by large organisations are often inconsistent in subtle ways with what the organisation is really doing on the ground, reflecting the outcomes of writing by committee, international negotiation or power-struggles on the one hand, and pragmatic responses to need on the other.

17   As with many bad ideas in economics, it can probably be tweaked to mitigate its worst aspects.

18   Colonial regimes sometimes used poll taxes in a similar way to force subsistence agriculturalists to work in plantation agriculture, similar to how archaic states taxed their subjects in precious metals even though they controlled the mines, so they could simply have confiscated all the money at source[22].

19   It is not the countries that become richer, it is the people in them. This is an important distinction when there is substantial inequality and the evaluation is made on aggregate data. It is likely to be just some of the people who become richer. Probably the ones who have least need for the money.

20   Accumulation of human capital is different from accumulation of finance capital because people have a sell-by-date when they retire, and a date of death after which they will not contribute to the economy. Finance capital can persist indefinitely, especially if a central bank resurrects it with a bailout when the markets collapse.

21   Though they may be less efficient than single-payer insurance systems in delivering a high quality of care.

22   Books about health economics often begin by explaining that the health sector experiences market failure, but this very term implies a contrast with market success, as if this holy grail might exist. The conditions for Pareto optimality to exist are complicated. In natural science we often use Occam's razor: the idea that a parsimonious model is preferable among competing models, in the absence of data. On this criterion the 'Stalin' model easily outcompetes the neoclassical economics one. There are only two conditions that need to be satisfied for the optimal system of distribution to be central allocation by a dictator – the dictator must be benevolent and hold complete information. During the cold war period neither condition held, so as with the neoclassical model none of the assumptions of the enthusiasts were valid. Turning to the empirical evidence, the time series of life expectancy from Russia suggests that rampant individualism (post 1989) justified by a neoclassical economic model, did not out-perform centralised planning in terms of its effect on life-expectancy (Figure 6).

23   Both bilateral assistance, and multilateral programs like the Global Fund[91] and GAVI[92].

24   Although studies of various measures of generosity find that in general poor people are more generous than the rich and high status[93].

25   People working in philanthropic foundations often seem to assume that best practice in giving away money is the same as best practice in accumulating it, even though the two activities are the opposite of each other. Maybe a psychologist looking would suggest reducing the stress involved in the accumulation process, resulting in less money to give away and hence less stress in the process of giving.

26   All billionaires should read the Ben Elton novel 'This Other Eden'[95] before making any plans for leaving planet Earth. Or maybe we would be better off if they don't read it.

27   Because much of it is covered with similar red laterite soils, and the people are mostly poor, black and all look the same to Europeans.

6. Health choices: the example of Insecticide Treated Nets

'The country is infested by swarms of mosquitoes ... everyone ... provides himself with a net, which during the day he uses for fishing, and at night fixes up round his bed, and creeps in under it before he goes to sleep. .... [the mosquitoes] do not even attempt to get through the net.'—Herodotus[97]

The book 'Effective altruism' [98] popularised the notion that evidence and reasoning might be used to determine the most effective ways to benefit others. Its advocates propose that it is more beneficial for people to use their existing skill sets to earn money, and then to give it way, rather than for them to retrain in something beneficial for the world that they might not be very good at.

Effective altruism has become a philosophy and social movement with a significant following among the small minority of people who consider themselves to be richer than they think they should be. One of the options for giving that is considered the most cost effective, and hence efficient, is to pay into programs that distribute insecticide treated mosquito nets (ITNs) for use against malaria in Africa.

Malaria has been one of the main killer diseases in the world throughout human history, though the fact that it is transmitted by mosquitoes was only established in the last decade of the 19th century[99]. People have always been irritated by mosquitoes, and the use of mosquito nets to protect against them was described in possibly the world's first history book[97], written by the ancient Greek historian Herodotus (see above for his description of their use in Egypt). The Egyptians do not appear to have thought this was a novel idea, so no-one knows when people started using mosquito nets to protect themselves from being bitten by mosquitoes. They have continued to be used throughout history.

When the World Health Organisation was founded after World War II, it was set the goal of eradicating malaria from the world by killing mosquitoes. The subsequent global malaria eradication campaign of 1955-69 got rid of malaria from much of the world mainly by insecticidal spraying of mosquito resting places[100] [1]. For some reason, it did not use mosquito nets[2]. When it became apparent that wall-spraying would not eliminate malaria from the African savannah or from tropical South Asia and South America, the rest of the world largely forgot about malaria[3].

During World War II several armies had tried out dipping mosquito nets in insecticide, which seemed to provide extra protection against malaria, and in the late 1980s researchers at the London School of Hygiene and Tropical Medicine, and the UK Medical Research council laboratories in The Gambia came up with the idea of using such nets treated with pyrethroids[4] to protect African children, the main victims of the disease. A small trial found that this prevented disease[102] another study found it reduced the numbers of infectious mosquitoes [103] and then a large comparison of villages with ITNs with villages without came up with the astonishing figure that they reduce child deaths by 63%[104]. At that time, it was not easy to find out how many children were dying from malaria, and researchers would casually cite a global estimate of 2.5 million per year[105] (equivalent to several Covid-19 pandemics). This was little more than a back-of-an-envelope calculation. Pedro Alonso's result[104] implied that most of these deaths could be averted by using a technology that cost about $5 per net. The first trial was followed up by other, better designed ones, that found that the proportion of all child deaths (not just malaria ones) that could be prevented by ITNs was a lower, but still very substantial[106-108], average of 17% [109].

Epidemiologists can be good at demonstrating what is good for our health but tend to adopt a subordinate role in policymaking. There was a caution about getting too excited about the potential of ITNs to impact malaria transmission, because of the demoralisation associated with the demise of the 1955-69 eradication program. For the first decade after the demonstration that ITNs work, there was also a general assumption that the pitifully small amounts of money available for malaria programs would not increase substantially, even though the amount of money required to buy ITNs for everyone was tiny in relation to the potential health effects. Table 1 presents both approximate values for the costs involved and some other economic statistics relating to the same time period, to help place these numbers in context.

Table 1. Some statistics of possible relevance to ITNs in Africa: (approximate values for the early 1990s).

African population	600 million
Required ITNs per person	0.5
Unit cost of ITN	$5
Lifetime of ITN	3 years
Global GDP	25 trillion
Percent GDP spent on military	3 %
Barbie dolls sold per year globally	20 million
Unit cost of Barbie	$25[5]

Derived values

Required ITNs per year	100	million
Annual cost of ITNs (cost of goods only)	$0.5	billions
Annual expenditure on Barbies[6]	$0.5	billions
Annual global military spend	$750	billions

Given that public health scientists did not control national budgets in either rich or poor countries, social marketing programs were set up to try to convince rural Africans to buy subsidised ITNs out of their meagre incomes [110]. This fitted into development ideologies that promote incorporation of subsistence agriculturalists into the market economy (Chapter 5) and related to that. The argument that people do not value things that they have not paid for, was used to argue against giving nets away. But since pregnant women and babies are the groups most vulnerable to malaria but have the least control over the purse-strings, programs were set up to give free ITNs to these groups[111][7]. The insecticide treatment would rapidly wash out of the original ITNs, so they needed to be retreated with sachets of insecticide. Retreatment rates were low. It took a further decade for nets that were persistently impregnated with insecticide (long-lasting) to be tested and widely available[112].

The original trials had involved giving ITNs to everyone, not just the people at high risk of disease and death, and when ITNs were being targeted to the youngest children only, some scientists were concerned that they might divert mosquitoes onto unprotected people[113][8]. It took some time for researchers to be convinced that, on the contrary, ITNs were protecting the rest of the community by killing mosquitoes that might otherwise have bitten someone else[115-117][9].

At a summit in Abuja in 2000, African governments had set themselves a target of protecting 60% of their populations with ITNs, but this would have gone nowhere but for a few influential individuals who realized that mass distribution of ITNs was both extremely cheap and would have an enormous health benefit. Firstly, Bill and Melinda Gates, via their foundation, started to spend money on malaria interventions, and after initially concentrating funding largely on malaria vaccines[10], began substantial funding of ITNs. Then Jeffery Sachs became a lobbyist for mass distribution of ITNs (Chapter 5).

Large scale distribution of long-lasting nets started in 2005[119], mostly funded by development assistance via the Global Fund Against Aids, Tuberculosis, and Malaria (GFATM)[91] (a multilateral fund initiated by the United Nations in 2001). Since then, GFATM has funded distribution of many hundreds of millions of ITNs (its headline in mid-2020 was that 131 million were distributed in 2018 alone). And WHO estimates that the death rate from malaria has fallen by about 60% compared to the turn of the 21st century, to about 400,000 deaths per year in 2019 [120]. Most of this effect has been achieved by ITNs[10].

This story of success, from the health perspective, flies in the face of a whole series of dogmas:

- The enthusiasts of unconstrained markets, like William Easterly, might see it as an example of the tyranny of experts[121] handing out ITNs willy-nilly, to the frustration of the markets, which would have preferred the money to be spent on Barbies. The handouts have created a market for ITNs, but this is not some Hayekian free-for-all. There are manufacturing plants across the globe, including China and Tanzania, but the market needs to be regulated and is regulated by the World Health

Organisation. The regulatory standards prevent the net market being dominated by cheap products from which the insecticide washes out, or which fall apart very quickly.

- The success contradicts the notion that development assistance is unhelpful or positively damaging in countries with bad governance [122].
- Jeffrey Sachs might believe that ITNs are building human capital, the workers of the future, but as we saw in Chapter 5, the ITNs are largely in the wrong places for that.
- Technology enthusiasts, who think the poor should be rescued by high technology from the North, might reflect on the quote from Herodotus and whether the ancient Egyptians ever held a patent.
- Those who believe that long-term interactions with local communities are essential before any outside idea will be accepted, should reflect on the fact that most people use mosquito nets, even if, or perhaps because they received them as a gift (Chapter 1). Nets are delivered by local subcontractors, without any need for any profound engagement with communities.

So, giving ITNs to everyone exposed to malaria seems like a very efficient way of improving health even if does not fit with various dogmas about development. Does the 'effective altruist' want to know more? The first thing s/he might want to do is to compare with other health interventions to which s/he might donate. This can be analysed in a straightforward way, by taking the ratio of deaths averted to how much it costs[11]. This is the cost-effectiveness ratio. If the comparison is just between different malaria interventions, then this might be good enough. Malaria (like Covid-19) makes many more people ill than need to be hospitalised, and of those that are hospitalised, about 90% survive. Some interventions (like improving hospital care) do not change how many people fall ill but do change how many of them die. In either case, as with Covid-19, what concerns us is people dying. An awful lot of people need to get a nasty fever before anyone is as bothered about fevers as they are about a single death.

ITNs are not the only intervention that can be used against malaria. The people making decisions about what to do about malaria in the countries where it remains a major problem (like the ministry of health), have many more considerations to weigh up than are summarised in a cost-effectiveness ratio[123]. They might be interested in how large their budget needs to be, or more likely how to spend a fixed budget. They also need to consider that what is feasible and works well in one place, may not be practicable somewhere else. So long as only one disease is being considered, though, these decisions need not be heavily value laden.

Things become much more complicated though, when more than one disease is in focus, and this is unavoidable when thinking about heath care, not prevention. At the health centres where the children with malaria are queueing for treatment with their mothers, there are also patients with pneumonia, skin infections, and parasitic worms.......

But the problem becomes thorny if the different options concern different diseases affecting people at different ages, and with different severity. A rather straightforward extension to counting deaths, is to count life-years. If a young child dies, it may lose eighty years of life, an elderly Covid-19 patient, perhaps four. Can simple arithmetic be used to simply count each child death as equivalent to twenty Covid-19 deaths? The decision theorists who work with such problems would mostly prefer to consider the quality of those years of life, which depends on all the emotional, social and physical aspects of our lives. To allow for this, the quality adjusted life-year (QALY) has been invented. Each year of life is given a weight depending on a measure of quality.

Each complication in this procedure adds more thorny questions. The QALY is used in decision making as an average across groups of patients or people at risk of disease, but underlying it are valuations that apply to individuals. If I am sick because I have a low income, am stressed by debts I cannot pay and an aggressive partner, does that mean that my life is worth less? The assessment of quality of life is complicated and has not been done in many places. If comparisons are made across countries, and issues of equity come to the fore so in international comparisons and low income countries, instead of the QALY, the disability adjusted life year (DALY)[124] is used as a standard measure in economic evaluations. The DALY is designed with the democratic intent that a healthy year of life counts the same for everyone, and the weighting of ill-health depends on which diseases a person is suffering from[12].

Should policy decisions about health (and by extension, about many other things) simply be made by doing calculations with QALYs and DALYs? The next two chapters ask the question of whether this is all that is needed to plot out a healthy future.

---

1   The mathematical model of George Macdonald[101] which implied that killing adult mosquitoes was likely to be the most effective way of reducing malaria transmission, was at the heart of the rationale for insecticide spraying, and for the design of the programs of which spraying was part.

2   Possibly because many people are prejudiced in favour of developing new technologies (such as malaria vaccines), even though it is often much more straightforward to improve the implementation of simpler, older technologies.

3   When it became apparent that Macdonald's model was an inadequate basis for planning malaria eradication, malaria scientists largely became deeply distrustful of mathematical modelling. An analogy would be if economic calculations that went beyond accountancy had been abandoned as a result of the Dutch tulip mania of the mid-seventeenth century.

4   Pyrethroid insecticides are chemically close to natural products and form the main class of insecticides for use indoors, since they are less harmful to humans than other pesticides.

5   Assuming a modest expenditure on add-ons.

6   It is presumably unrealistic to expect military expenditure, intended for killing people, to be repurposed to prevent children from dying. However, since the amount of money involved is close to the total the Barbie owners are used to dealing with, they might have been expected to be more sympathetic to the plight of other children.

7   This is rather like protecting the elderly and frail while leaving the Covid-19 virus to spread in the rest of society, an idea floated early in the current pandemic.

8   There were also concerns that protection with ITNs might defer the first infections that babies receive until the age when they had lost the immunological protection gained via their mothers[114]. These issues were addressed in further careful research.

9   Some people argued that ITNs should be treated as a 'public good' like public parks or law enforcement, which are generally paid for out of taxation[118]. This argument was confusing as it was the richer people who bought ITNs and protected the others, and there was no prospect of community wide pooling of resources via local taxation.

10   Vaccines are extraordinarily efficient interventions against some pathogens, especially viruses like measles, whooping cough, mumps, and rubella, that used to kill or disable enormous numbers of children. Antivaccine campaigners are mostly too young to remember these nasty infections that used to blight our childhoods. As with Covid-19 social distancing would be the best alternative to vaccines for controlling these directly transmitted viral infections. The antivaccine lobby might want to think twice about being responsible for more lockdowns if these viruses come back. Malaria vaccines represent a much greater technological challenge than vaccines against the former viral diseases of childhood. Where it is a possibility, killing mosquitoes is generally a more efficient alternative to either vaccines or lockdowns.

11   It is not trivial to establish the cost as this should include both the price of goods, and the various expenses involved in delivering nets, including the costs of organising this.

12   As well as disability weighting the inventors of the DALY[124] initially weighted years differently by age. Sometimes discounting is used to allow for the fact that we care more about the immediate future, than the long term, which in any case is uncertain.

7. Your Money or Your Life: where Decision Theory falls Sick and Loses its Mind

"It is health that is real wealth and not pieces of gold and silver." —Mohandas Gandhi

In a stereotype of the gothic novel, "Your money or your life" is the phrase used by a highwayman when he holds up a stagecoach at gunpoint. As a victim you suddenly appear to be faced with a profound existential decision between payment or death. But of course, it is no choice at all. Dead, your money is worth nothing to you and the robber would no doubt take it anyway. So, it seems rather obvious that you should take out your wallet and hand it over. Even then, you might still be shot[1].

There is an analogy between this hold-up scenario and how decisions are made about health and well-being. Sometimes, when it appears that choices must be made between unpleasant alternatives, there really is no alternative available. Sometimes what should be obvious is hidden by the ways we are trained to frame the question. There is no real dilemma in choosing between money and life. Like WH Auden's line from 'September 1, 1939', '*We must love one another or die* '. Auden himself subsequently pointed out that we must die anyway.

The kinds of questions posed in Chapter 6 are about life and death. It can be hard to address them, but they are questions about efficiency (usually some variant on how to get the biggest health impact from a fixed amount of money). That might be a complicated question to answer, but it does not require us to make comparisons where there may be a trade-off with between lives and something else. Yet many decisions require exactly that. The most frequently used health economic approaches for deciding which strategy to adopt belong to a set of approaches called rational choice theory that in effect use monetary values for the value of life. These values, referred to as the willingness-to-pay represent the highest value (ceiling ratio) that a 'rational' entity should be prepared to pay to save one unit of health[2].

These entail either estimating the health benefit of the intervention program (in the case that it is intended to improve health) or the monetary benefit in the case that the intervention it is intended to make cost savings, but only if the health consequences of the savings are small[126]. If we specify the willingness-to-pay, then simple algebra relates these quantities. The decision rule is effectively the same but the willingness-to-pay has performed an almost magical role in transforming a Cost Effectiveness Analysis (as described in Chapter 6) into a cost benefit analysis . The idea is that if someone or some organisation is willing to pay a defined amount of money to avert one QALY then the health effects, then the health and economic effects can be added up on the same scale[3]

Effectively a cost-benefit analysis treats the willingness-to-pay as the value of life. Many people are shocked when they first encounter cost-benefit analysis applied to health. There is something shocking about assigning a monetary value to life. There are various approaches that aim to determine value of life by finding out how much money people think their own or other peoples' lives are worth, ranging from the very simple and obviously naïve, to the technically sophisticated and challenging to implement. The simplest one is to ask someone (or ask a lot of people, and then calculate an average). Imagine the following phone conversation[4]:

"Hello, I'm a health decision expert, I'm calling to ask how much your granny is worth."

"What? Are you crazy or something?"

"I just want you to put a value on your granny. Like, is it $20,000 or more than that?"

"I think you're a hit man. Or maybe a cold caller whose been hired by an unemployed hitman to sign people up. If you were really something to do with health, you wouldn't ask stupid questions like that."

"Well, let's put it this way. Is she worth more than you?"[5]

"I really don't want to answer that because I might get arrested. But just between you and me, if the choice were between the two of us, I'd say she was worth maybe...... $10."[6]

"I don't believe you. What if the choice was between losing your granny, who is old, and will die soon anyway, and wiping out a young person you don't know? Sort of like in a horror film where people are playing video games, that involve wiping out avatars by clicking on them, except that the other players are killed for real. Come to think of it, if I could convince you that it was for real, that would be a good way of getting answers out of you. We could set up the software so that you had to kill one or other, or at least you thought you did."

"I think that would put me off video games for life."

"What if the choice was between winning a million dollars betting on football, at odds of 3:2, and forcing your granny to play Russian roulette.[7]"

"Pass."

"I'd like you to answer a different kind of question. If you were in a funicular, like the one coming down from Gerschnialp to Engelberg in the Swiss Alps, say, and the cable breaks, there's no brake and you are zooming towards a place on the line where it branches. You have a handle which determines which way to go either to the left, or to the right, but .....[8]"

"Yes?"

"There are two sheep on the left-hand track, and three on the right hand one. "

"What about the cabin coming up towards me. I guess I would try to avoid it."

"Forget about that."

"A bit unlikely, but OK, I suppose I would wipe out the two sheep."

"What if it was 100 sheep on one track and your granny on the other?"

"You've got me now. I suppose I would just put my hands over my eyes and take pot-luck.[9]"

"OK. You're refusing to answer. But every day decisions must be made that require us to put a value on life. I'll just have to watch what you do, and work out how much you really value your granny, from things like whether you are more likely to get out of bed to check she is alright when the alarm beeps to say she might be having a heart attack and you should check up on her, or when you get a text saying you won two million dollars in the lottery providing you pick it up before 9 a.m.[10]."

This decision theorist is clearly a loose cannon who is mixing different methodologies aiming at answering a very difficult question[11]. There is no particular reason why the answers given to any of his questions should provide some hidden ideal value of life, because it is the questioner who insists that there must be such a thing, not the person answering the question. Most of us never face any choices anything like the ones described above in reality. If we are unfortunate enough to be trapped by them, we use heuristics, rough and ready decision rules that are not guaranteed to be optimal[61, 133], and these will operate differently depending on the framing of the scenarios from which data are collected.

The suggestion that the problem can be solved with a surveillance camera in the bedroom substantially underestimates what the health economist needs to do. Revealed preferences [134] is generally the preferred approach but requires analysis of substantial amounts of data on how people have spent their money and the choices they have made. When this is done, it turns out that this method will assign a value to life that is more than other methods[135] and far more than any health system is prepared to pay.

It seems at first sight plausible that the preferences that are revealed in our choices correspond to our values. Or at least it might have seemed plausible to economists until these assumptions were overturned by behavioural economics and prospect theory[61, 69]. Often, if asked, we may even admit to choosing the wrong thing. Moreover, there is no way of validating revealed preferences against anything else, so it has been claimed that it is a tautological fallacy. See, *inter alia*, the critiques by Amartya Sen[136-138].

Despite all these criticisms, rational choice theory has been increasingly used in resource allocation decisions in the health system. Although the UK National Health Service was originally built on socialist principles that precluded market logic (e.g. [139]) the UK is where this is most pervasive, since it was institutionalised within the National Health Service with the establishment of the National Institute for Health and Care Excellence (NICE). NICE uses willingness-to-pay thresholds of £20,000 - £30,000 per QALY[140], and the UK used to allocate roughly the right amount of money to pay for this, though the best estimate of what was actually paid in the UK (in 2008) was £12,900 per QALY. In this field other countries are often analysed by reference to the UK.

WHO say willingness-to-pay thresholds should be between 100-300% of the national GDP per capita. This is intended to reflect affordability[134], but what is actually paid is much less than the per capita GDP in most countries[141]. No-one other than affluent people paying from their own resources, will pay for the interventions that WHO is recommending. These thresholds are intended to be valid only within a setting, not for international comparisons and by presenting them WHO is aiming to mobilize donor support to expand access to better medicines for all.

The interventions that are cost-effective but unaffordable are likely to be the most sensible ones for donors to spend their money on. Even then, linking the recommended threshold to GDP means that a life appears to have a much lower value in a poor country than in a rich country. Few would argue publicly that a Congolese is worth less than a Swiss, though in practice the way we treat the Congolese suggests that national-level willingness-to-pay thresholds may indeed be indicative of a disturbing inequity in the way people are valued.

Statistical value of life is promoted as a bureaucratic metric allowing practical comparisons for use in budgets, between sectors of the economy and different outcomes within sectors. Within the health sector everything might be reduced to QALYs or DALYs. A cost benefit analysis is used if factors from multiple sectors are being considered[12].

Proponents of decision-making based on willingness-to-pay may argue these decisions are only life-and-death in statistical terms, so willingness-to-pay is not the same as value of life. Individuals personally affected by the decisions might see this differently. But the across the world at this moment many instantaneous life or death choices are being made at the individual level, because of triage[13]. Triage is the practice of dividing patients up according to whether they are likely to die anyway; whether they will recover without very much medical attention, or whether they are in the intermediate category where appropriate care would make all the difference. During the Covid-19 pandemic patients are being triaged to make sure that those who are likely to be saved are assigned the limited numbers of ventilators available. In some countries, patients who were living in care homes before the pandemic, and who are likely to be very old and have severe underlying conditions like dementia, come into the first category.

The concept of triage was invented by a French surgeon during the Napoleonic Wars[143]. In battlefield situations immediate choices need to be made instantly about which of the casualties to try to save. The same thing can happen in emergency rooms. After the pandemic there may be a lot of people who will know what it feels like to make these decisions. Most jurisdictions have developed procedures to guide these decisions[144] but in the crisis situations that are depicted in the media it is unlikely that a carefully considered decision aligned with the fine-print of the guidelines can be made in each case. Some of the physicians may indeed be assigning numerical values to patients and abandoning the ones with low values but that is just because, as the health decision expert implied before the phone was slammed down, faced with that situation you have to do something.

In normal times, when there is time to make health policy decisions at leisure, there are ethics boards to consult over challenging decisions like these. Many scientists experience ethics boards simply as a force for bureaucratic obstruction, that makes it hard to do as much research as you need to do, in order to keep your publication output high enough to obtain a position with a stable salary. In principle though, ethics boards are there to ensure that physicians and researchers adhere to a set of rules that have achieved broad consensus. These rules are those of medical ethics, founded in deontological philosophy, which maintains that whether an action is right or wrong depends on a series of rules, rather than on its consequences. To deontologists the utilitarian philosophy of rational choice theory is a sort of relic of 19th century philosophers (Bentham and John Stuart Mill[14]) whom a philosophy undergraduate might learn about before moving on to serious stuff.

Measures of health differ fundamentally from money since health in this sense is not abstract. Most starkly whether someone dies or not is clearly marked in a way that could be apparent to an alien from another planet. Monetary value is not. The alien could understand monetary values only in the context of the whole system of exchange that determines what can be bought with the money.

The use of willingness to pay implies that it is rational to make health decisions using calculations based on quantitatively defined utilities, effectively equating so much consumption of consumer items to a life, or to a different health state. This would be completely invisible to the alien who might reasonably judge that whatever was going on was certainly not rational. But rational choice theorists have pre-empted the use of the word 'rational' making it difficult to argue that they are irrational. Fast forward however, to the Covid-19 pandemic (Chapter 9), and we see that almost the only politicians arguing there is a simple trade-off between lives and cost are Donald Trump and his friends. Most of the world thinks there is much more to these choices. Chapter 8 continues the exploration of why this is the case.

Economic man (Chapter 4) is keen on rational choice theory but is particularly susceptible to epidemic disease. This is because he is defined as being independent of his fellow economic man [15]. Unsurprisingly, he is uncomfortable with viral spread of preferences......... [16], but he has not given up "You might have given me a bruising," he cries," But you will need me in the end. You can't pay infinity for a life, because of scarcity….".

1   There is an alternative: to resist. This choice would probably not be advised by an expert in travel security. However, by adopting a dominant role the robber framed the possibilities in a way that made it unlikely that you would think of this messy option in the heat of the moment. It probably makes sense to hand over the money and hope for the best. By producing a gun in the first place the robber (or rather the novel's author) has also framed the situation as a conflict, where someone is bound to lose out.

2   Revealed preference approaches can be applied irrespective of whether the unit of health is the illness episode, death, QALY, or DALY so they are used to calculate quality and disability weightings for QALYs and DALYs[125]. The same objections apply to this use of revealed preferences as to their use for valuing life itself.

3   Cost benefit analysis cannot be a generally valid approach for guiding social choices, since repugnant outcomes like slavery (see e.g. [22]) are not excluded and it can lead to inequality. Ways of engaging with issues of fairness and equality have been proposed by Rawl's[127], and via Nussbaum and Sen's capabilities approach[46]. A key result is Arrow's Impossibility Theorem[128] which broadly means that in the general case there is no right answer. Not a problem easily dealt with during a pandemic.

4   The specific questions used in the example, which is exaggerated to try to make it entertaining, are obviously absurd. However, questions with the same logical structure as those in this bizarre exchange are indeed used to place values on life for different purposes.

5   The answers to any of these questions would probably be different if the respondent was being asked about his/herself rather than granny.

6   This corresponds to the approach of contingent valuation, which uses surveys asking people to directly report their willingness-to-pay for specified outcomes.

7   This refers to the use of standard gambles to try to elicit a value for human life. This example is not of course very standard, but you might get the idea. Standard gamble questions involve a choice between different health states with different probabilities. These are often used to obtain measures of quality of life (QALY)[129]. Implicitly this requires that the person answering the questions understands probabilities (apart from anything else).

8   This is an approach for eliciting value judgements used by ethicists, frequently referred to as a 'trolley' problem[130]. The value of this approach for eliciting any practically useful information is questionable because the scenario is almost unimaginable. I have located it in a specific place to make it just that bit more plausible. The questions could be posed either as 'What should you do?' or 'What would you do?'

9   This may indicate that this is an indifference point in the stated preference approach, or more likely that the respondent does not want to think about the question. It is unlikely to be a useful way of eliciting information about serious conditions or death. It is more likely to be used to elicit preferences about possibly less emotive issues like parking policy (but is sometimes used in health studies [131])

10   This is the revealed preferences approach, considered by its proponents to be un-problematical because it is possible to observe the real choices that people really make, which avoids the problem that what people say may be quite different from what they do. It does assume that humans make decisions by calculating based on a consistent utility function i.e. that consumer behaviour is rational whereas opting out of the rat-race is not[132], contrary to the conclusions of most reflective people. Consumer behaviour is of course influenced by advertisers and deceitful 'influencers' whose activities open up another can of worms.

11   S/he is probably a PhD student doing a pilot study for a thesis that is still waiting for ethical approval.

12   Cost benefit analysis consequently has an insidious use as a political tool for advocating whatever happens to be the fashion of the time. As a young political activist in Edinburgh, Scotland, in the 1980s I was involved in the campaign against extension of the motorway from Glasgow into the centre of the city. The advocates of the plan cited the cost benefit analysis that they had commissioned to show that the experts thought it was a good idea. (The defeat of this road plan was one of the few victories we had during the 1980s. It was not done by critiquing the cost benefit analysis, though it occurred to me at the time that 'someone' should have done this). My future wife was working with the transport planning department round about the same time. Every major decision was informed by a cost benefit analysis.

A couple of decades later, a tramway was constructed along the same route through the west of Edinburgh. Very likely a different firm of consultants were hired to do the cost benefit analysis. They presumably adjusted the list of factors included in the main analysis, treating a different sub-set as externalities (i.e. effects not important enough to be worth putting a number on). I suspect the first cost benefit analysis treated the health effects of vehicle emissions [142], as an externality not important enough to try to cost. The idea of including effects on climate of CO_2 release wouldn't even have been laughed at in the 1980s.

13   Triage is the French word for separate. The most frequent usage I have encountered is in relation to sorting out garbage into things that can be recycled and those that are put in the undifferentiated waste.

14   In contrast to Bentham, John Stuart Mill thought you could use the sum total of happiness as a measure of utility, which is a short step from asking the question how much does it cost to buy so much happiness i.e. $$$= happiness, which leads directly to the illusions of consumerism.

15   I have never read of economic woman. Perhaps she committed suicide to avoid going through all the logical torment. Since economic man does not form emotional bonds, he also has problems with sex.

16   Perhaps it is possible to incorporate non-linear spread of preferences across a contact network into a formal model of revealed preferences. Someone should try it. It might keep him/her off the streets for a long time, where s/he could otherwise be causing trouble. Alternatively, s/he could log on to Facebook and make friends with all the other people already implementing a similar model in cyberspace, wondering why they are plagued with posts that they don't want to see.

8. The last gasp of economic man

"We know how this ends. You're going to die and so will everyone you love......But that's not how we live our lives. Humans might be in unique possession of the knowledge that our existence is essentially meaningless, but we carry on as if in ignorance of it." —Will Storr[15].

Rational choice theorists face severe problems when faced with mortality [89].

While writing these essays I have been acutely aware that many readers will be objecting that a long-life is not the same as a good one (in any sense of the word good). We value more things that just how long we live. Hence attempts to improve on life-expectancy by allowing for disability and quality of life, using measures such as the DALY, QALY or the number of healthy life-years. These already lead into the murky area of assessing the relative value of different life-states (Chapter 7).

Some of the problems with death are mathematical. Up to now, this book has frequently resorted to the hard numbers of life-expectancy, using this term as shorthand for life-expectancy at birth, the average number of years that a new born would live, if the chances of dying at each age remain the same as they were in its year of birth. This is not how long a baby is likely to live. If it lives in a period of increasing capabilities, it will probably live longer than its life expectancy at birth. If it is born in a world with imminent wars and epidemics, it will die sooner. If a single number is to be used to measure how healthy is a population then life-expectancy works well partly because death is unambiguous. Apart from a few comatose patients, it is clear when someone dies, and so it is possible to make meaningful comparisons of this statistic between places and over the millennia.

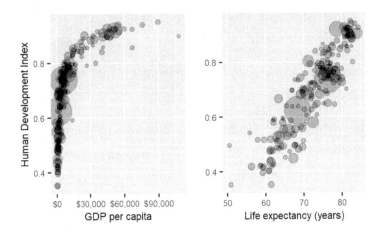

Figure 13. Human Development Index by GDP and Life Expectancy[1]

Our capabilities are not just a matter of being alive, so the United Nations Development Program, has developed a statistic, the Human Development Index(HDI)[145], that tries to do better than using life expectancy (or healthy life-years, or QALYs) as a measure of health and wellbeing (Figure 13). This takes as inputs data on life expectancy, GDP, and education to calculate for each country a number that in principle might vary between zero and one.

The HDI overcomes some of the limitations of GDP as a measure of well-being, With GDP, every dollar counts equally, whether held by a billionaire or a pauper, though the value of the pauper's dollar, in terms of human well-being is obviously greater. Like life-expectancy, HDI has an upper limit. But it is not obvious that HDI helps to overcome the deficiencies of life-expectancy. As should be clear from Chapters 3 and 5 both high GDP and educational attainment lead to high life-expectancy, so it seems like double-counting to create a measure that considers these as valuable in themselves, as well as contributing via their effects on life expectancy. Moreover, if HDI is treated as a target for development programs, it suffers like all targets that only approximate what is the real objective, from gaming of the system. Instead of working to improve health, which is what is ultimately desired, it incentivises irrelevant improvements in imperfect measures. For instance, educational attainment feeds into the HDI. Education statistics might be improved by grade inflation, or by reclassifying schools as universities, neither of which really contribute to wellbeing.

Regulation by targets assumes that priorities can really be targeted, with what is measured adequately representing everything that is desired, so that what is left out does not matter.[146], Given that HDI is very strongly correlated with life-expectancy anyway (right hand side of Figure 13), and that HDI is generally only available at national level, and for a limited historical period, it is not clear that it has any advantages as a way of measuring the well-being of a population. Life expectancy is also harder to game, but even extending life at all costs is not always desirable. The calculus of QALYs has problems with end-of-life decisions over palliative care[2], euthanasia, or assisted suicide. Albert Einstein had a point when he said: *"Not everything that counts can be measured, and not everything that can be measured counts"*[3].

The inventors of the DALY originally proposed age-weighting of life-years and discounting of the future[124], but any way of doing this is obviously questionable and these elements exposed the arbitrariness of weighting time. A fundamental problem with any time-weighting of our lives is that we do not value every moment equally. A point captured by the poet Wordsworth[148]:

"There are in our existence spots of time,
That with distinct pre-eminence retain
A renovating virtue.....,
...... by which pleasure is enhanced,
That penetrates, enables us to mount,
When high, more high, and lifts us up when fallen."

We value events, not merely some average quality of extended periods of time in our life. The brain recalls specific moments, specific achievements, and failures, not in general as periods, weighted by how long they lasted, but as events. There are critical events, which themselves may have lasted only moments (accidents, deaths, decisions), but which colour life disproportionately[4]. In our memories, events stand out disproportionately relative to their duration, the extension of long periods of repetition, tedium, less so[5].

Naïve utilitarianism hits its limits not only at the end of life, but also at the beginning. It has nothing useful to say about contraception. The desirability, or otherwise, of reproduction is a field of contention with reproductive rights campaigners caught in the middle between Malthusians, and pronatalist politicians (who want to see their own ethnicity or nationality growing in numbers), and religions with analogous agendas.

The logic of calculus of utilities means that we should always assign a positive utility to each new human[6] (putting the utilitarians in the same camp as the Catholic church). This flies in the face of the presumptions of most progressives. Many of the world's governments have pronatalist policies, at the same time as limiting immigration. Dog-whistle politicians promoting pronatalism at the same time as excluding immigrants, seem to tap into deep seated attitudes that would have made sense in the Palaeolithic societies described in Chapter 1. They want to see more people like themselves, and fewer of those who are different.

Let us return to the Gerschnialp funicular in Chapter 7, poised in mid-descent with granny on one line, and a flock of sheep on the other. It seems obvious that many people would be torn between what they feel they ought to value, and what they do in fact value (perhaps a better example than the sheep could be used to illustrated this). Just as many of us would like to see natural environments with fewer human impacts, while simultaneously acknowledging that there are too many people in the world. George Monbiot enjoyed rewilded environments in Slovenia, while recognising that these areas are empty of humans only because of genocide during and after the 2nd world war[149]. Many of us would like to live in a world that was less cluttered with other humans even if we are liberal minded and like to have friends who are different from ourselves.

More generally the ways we make life and death decisions defy formal analysis. They are the stuff of literature. There is more on this in Shakespeare than will ever be found in the pages of economics texts. It is a myth that we will ever be comfortable with decisions made about this on technical economic criteria.

The inadequacy of the utilitarian perspective is most obvious when it comes to the ways we think about death. Death, and the circumstances around it, are especially important to us, however much we avoid talking about them. There is no plausible way of trading off pain, regret, guilt against each other. When we think about the implications of different ways of dying, we cannot obtain first-hand information from the dead. Those around someone who dies, their friends, their relatives, react in different ways conditioned by religion, by their socialisation, and by their connection to the deceased.

A visit to a medieval cathedral, packed with tombs and memorials, serves as a reminder that for most of human existence, manifestations of death were ubiquitous. Death, mostly from infectious disease, was unpredictable and could happen at any age[7]. This is the context in which the world's major religions arose, and a big part of their social function of religion was, and remains, to deal with the emotional mayhem associated with the end of life. The extreme rationalists of the French Revolution invented the guillotine[8] but the very idea that death can be treated so mechanically stirs up all the passions it was meant to cut off.

Funerary traditions from the prehistoric until the present contradict the assumption that what matters about a person ends with their death. We care about implementing the wishes of the dead (for instance as expressed in wills) and there are whole industries focusing on catering to individualised funeral practices. Religious traditions that believe in an afterlife earned either by deeds or thoughts, offer an approach to rational behaviour at variance with economic man. This is at the price of irrational belief, but so-called rationalists also consider their intellectual legacy to matter[9], and perhaps surprisingly, even the disposal of their bodies.

The civilisations of the past, from Egypt, Taj Mahal, to the Yucatan, have left an impression that they were obsessed with death, since the most durable structures they left were memorials to the dead. The similarities between Athens and Chichén Itzá hint at universals that likely go back further than humanity itself. When the conquistadors brought their version of European culture to the Americas, they found monumental architecture and awe of religion nearer to their own, than are either to liberal values of the 21st century. Europeans, from Ancient Greece and Rome, until the Victorian era, were no different.

The tourist guides and histories suggest it was the piety of the rulers that gave us all those monuments, but a little reflection tells us that it was rather their scepticism about the afterlife. Had they really believed the propaganda of their priests they would have had no need to leave great buildings on this earth. Rather they feared that without memorials in stone, for all their earthly power when alive, in death they would turn to nothing more than the same kind of dust and mould as would their millions of despised subjects. Like the meek, they would inherit nothing.

Are we to believe, these were all cultures morbidly obsessed with death, or that we are the odd ones-out? For the last 75 years In the industrialised world, death of all but the oldest has become infrequent (Chapter 2), the war memorials have been accumulating moss, and it is easy to forget that death could happen any time. Modern humans have few qualms about dispossessing Tutankhamun and more and more we discretely burn our dead and scatter their ashes anonymously and democratically. But we can never escape from mortality, and the fact that it makes a mockery of every attempt to make the world truly rational.

It is an easy step from these observations to conclude that most people are irrational most of the time, but this is not the same as failing to comply with a discredited model of rationality. Economic man is not rational either. Where is the rationality in spending our lives computing marginal financial benefits of small transactions, when in the end it is all for nothing? The notion of economic self-interest fails in the face of our mortality. How can it be rational to cumulate wealth beyond what we will ever spend?

Economic man, no longer having a stake in the matter, would not mind if his relatives tear up his will as soon as the ventilator is switched off. He agrees with the actor Dan Aykroyd that "*if a man dies with a single penny still sitting in the bank, he's a fool.*". He never cared about his descendants or about the world they will live in. Many of his supporters though, would think him irresponsible for this and are aghast at the thought of inheritance taxes[10].

1   Bubbles correspond to different countries with bubble area proportional to population. Based on free material from gapminder.org, CC-by license[36].

2   Perhaps partly explaining why palliative care in the UK has traditionally been largely supported by charities[147], rather than mainly by the National Health Service.

3   There is a substantial literature on the perverse incentives created by performance targets of one kind or another, and an enormous amount of target-setting by people who ignore that literature. This is not least in the international development world, with Millennium Development Goals, Sustainable Development Goals. Programs should generally be evaluated using quantities that were not set as targets, since gaming of the targets does not affect non-target measures.

4   Who are we to say that Nero was mad for when Rome burnt, or that the audience were crazy when they stopped to listen to the band on the Titanic? If you must die, why not savour the opportunity, if you have it, of first participating in one of the moments forts of history?

5   Perhaps one of the most telling behavioural economics findings is that the last part of an experience can dominate recall of the overall occurrence. People who put their hands for a period in uncomfortably hot water, report that the experience was less unpleasant if it was followed by an additional period with their hands in slightly less uncomfortably hot water[61].

6   The philosopher John Broome proposes ways of factoring the number of people into aggregate utility calculations, so that each additional person adds some amount of utility. An idea that conjures up imaginings of a dystopia where philosophers are conducting wild trolley experiments to deal with the problem of natural resource constraints.

7   Nowadays in wealthy countries, almost all deaths are in the elderly, but the proportion of people who die every year is not so much lower than in poorer countries. Death has been banished to retirement homes and hospitals.

8   The guillotine was invented as a humane alternative to other forms of execution used in the 18th century.

9   The founder of utilitarianism, Jeremy Bentham, who died in 1832, left instructions for his body to be first dissected, and then permanently preserved as an "auto-icon" (or self-image), which would be his memorial. The auto-icon remains on public display in University College London. It is hard to see that it has much utility. Perhaps Bentham imagined himself having the last laugh by trapping the funeral directors, whose business depends on defiance of his philosophy, into incurring an infinite expense by maintaining the auto-icon in perpetuity. The ones who were his contemporaries might have taken this personally. Subsequent generations of funeral directors might complain of post-mortem rent seeking. If anyone with a Ouija board has been in touch with Bentham, please let us know whether he is still enjoying the joke.

10 Biologists have argued that we are not so much selfish individuals but rather agents of our selfish genes[150], which we share with relatives. The notion of inclusive fitness thus provides an adaptationist evolutionary rationale for why humans want to pass wealth to future generations. This does not mean that large scale inherited wealth is either inevitable or socially desirable. Rational choice theory can also be extended to include preferences for where wealth will go after death, but the people alive in the future might legitimately object to their lives being constrained by the preferences of people who are long gone.

9. Economic man buried by a Chance Pandemic

"we must not return to normal because normal was the problem in the first place" —graffiti in Hong Kong.

Hardly anyone across the world can have been untouched by the Covid-19 pandemic, and there will ultimately no doubt be vast archives of books, films, blogs, recording the perspectives of different people, and what were the specifics of the event as they experienced it. This chapter does not attempt a summary of our experiences of the pandemic. Rather it explores how the themes of earlier chapters: fundamental elements of human psychology stemming from our pre-history described in Chapter 1, psychosocial effects on health (Chapter 3), our attitudes to mortality (Chapter 8) and chance events, have exposed the hollowness of the economic models that have dominated policy making in much of the world.

I feel like I have re-entered the realm of the unexpected[1]. Like almost everyone I was taken by surprise by the pandemic.[2] I did not have the same excuses as most, since by profession I am an infectious disease modeller. I was not much surprised that it happened, nor by the scale of the mortality, but I was surprised by the political response to it. When there were still only a few cases in Europe, a colleague suggested that it could cause the next economic crash. I was sceptical: I still thought the next global crash would most likely be caused by overvaluation of social media connection data held by Silicon Valley. Within a few weeks I was proven wrong. In Europe, politician after politician pointed out that the draconian lockdown and quarantine measures were a matter of life and death. "This is not a time for ideology or orthodoxy......" explained UK chancellor Rishi Sunak representing a political party that has presided over measurable declines in life-expectancy.[3]

Every year 50 million people or so die in the world, many of them from avoidable causes, and so someone wanting to argue that the lockdowns are overreaction is likely to compare the number of Covid-19 deaths with the background mortality from other causes or with historical epidemics, like those summarised in Chapter 1 or the 1918 Spanish Influenza (Chapter 2). The final death toll will clearly be nothing like that of 1918-19. If conservatively we assume the Spanish flu killed 1% of the population,[4] that would be over 80,000 people in contemporary Switzerland. If the Covid-19 epidemic were concentrated over 10 weeks, that would be 8000 deaths per week which is way off the top of the chart. The modeller, Christian Althaus, came up with a 'worst case scenario' of 30,000 deaths for Switzerland at the start of the epidemic, before anything was done to control it[153].

Those of us working in public health statistics are used to throwing around large numbers, and 30,000 seems large, but not enormous in that context[5]. This is less than half the total number of deaths in Switzerland in a normal year. We are also used to public health threats being ignored. This one was not ignored.

What was different?

Globally, economists' and politicians' reactions have varied. At one end of the spectrum are those associated with the Trump regime, whose reaction to the pandemic has been to argue that saving grannies is just not worth any disruption of the economy (for instance[154]), noting that the victims are predominantly the old and disabled who are no longer economically active, and don't have long to live anyway. A back-of-the-envelope cost effectiveness analysis, like one reported for Switzerland [155] suggests that government expenditure per QALY saved is way more than the highest WHO recommended threshold willingness-to-pay. This ignores the deep-rooted importance of kinship in human psychology (Chapter 1). 21st century humans are uncomfortable with having banished granny to a care home (because that was what post-industrial lifestyles required). We are not about to add an accusation that we treated her as expendable. Most politicians, at least in Europe, have the humanity to sense this too.

Most critically though, as an explanation for political reactions, epidemics trigger a perfect storm of anxiety. Behavioural economists have shown that we have strong preferences to cling on to what we have (the endowment effect), in this case our lives. We are strongly averse to risks, and when the risk is death, we would do almost anything to avoid it. Whatever the utility that a decision theorist assigns to my life, I am likely to think it is on the low side, and whatever the stakes, there are few takers for Russian roulette.

Few people alive in industrialised countries have experienced anything like this before[6]. The last major smallpox epidemic in Europe was in Yugoslavia in 1972. The few living survivors of the 1918 influenza, were small children at the time. This was concurrent with the World War I, when people in most of Europe had already spent four years getting used to friends and family dying in the war, so they probably experienced less of an endowment effect.

In the early stages of an epidemic, the risk has a further characteristic that adds to the collective anxiety. The risk itself is essentially unknown[7]. Acute uncertainty is a recognised cause of severe stress [156]. Uncertainty about uncertainty is doubly stressful. Along with the excitement of the challenge, this fear of the unknown may partly explain why, during early stages of the epidemic, an enormous number of people were developing mathematical models of Covid-19. Outbreak modelling is a large part of what infectious disease modellers are asked to do, but it is fraught with guesswork and technical challenges. Why do so many presume they can do better than the others? Many people who had previously shown no interest in modelling infectious disease, were intently rediscovering variants of the Susceptible Infectious Resistant (SIR) model, originally developed by Kermack and McKendrick in 1927[157]. Unfortunately for anyone seeking a quiet life, each new epidemic, HIV, BSE, Swine-flu SARS, Ebola, Covid-19 has a different ecology. A newbie, dabbling in this field will most likely rediscover measles.

Humans continually face new epidemic diseases, each with different ecologies[8] and even when the biology has been translated into mathematics, there is profound uncertainty early on about how much of it is the risk to public health, and what should be done to reduce this, because hardly any data are available[9]. Researchers were initially under enormous pressure to turn around results at unheard off timelines. because interventions early in the epidemic can be decisive[10]. As epidemics progress, the uncertainties become less, the possibilities of what might happen are being gradually reduced, but the uncertainty will only disappear when the pandemic is over.

At the level of governments there must have been a snowball effect. With the internet buzzing with lies, rumours and half-truths, the approaches to containment and suppression, once adopted by one country were transmitted like an infectious agent themselves, legitimately because of the need to move quickly, but irrespective of much analysis of collateral damage or assessment of feasibility. Once one European state closed its borders and introduced a lockdown, it would have been hard for the next one not to do the same. Meanwhile both fear of the disease itself, and the lockdowns that were introduced in response, were associated with panics, reminiscent of those caused by the medieval plagues.

In many people the anxiety associated with all this uncertainty and rapid change translated into panic. Stressed people are more likely to believe conspiracy theories[159], and many bizarre stories emerged during the pandemic[11]. Noticing coincidences is a recognised symptom of stress-induced mania and possibly accounts for many strange elements of our culture[12]. One such widely observed coincidence is that Covid-19, initially at least, disproportionately infected the exact demographic group who are in power. Climate shaming could not touch the politicians who have been leading us to hell in a frenzy of globalisation, but Covid-19 does. It struck the most mobile first. It disproportionately kills the baby-boomer generation who have led the world into an ecological mess. If it does not kill them it is burning up their savings, so Trump may believe it has been designed to wipe out his own base (diabolical intelligent design, or as Trumpians suggest, the Chinese Conspiracy). This is a clear example of confirmation bias or the prosecutor's fallacy[13]. Diseases that disproportionately wipe out poor people in remote places kill more people but just do not get in the news. In most of the world Covid-19 has received much greater media attention than did the HIV epidemic even at its peak when AIDS was untreatable. 32 million people died of AIDS[160] between the start of the epidemic and the end of 2018,, way more than will die of Covid-19. This was traumatizing in southern Africa and in the gay community in the North but was perceived as a niche issue elsewhere. In that instance some of religious felt superior and proclaimed the virus to be the wrath of God. With Covid-19, the religious were often at the heart of local spread of the epidemic, be they Muslims in Malaysia or the Protestants in Mulhouse[161]. That is another coincidence that should be discounted.

Epidemics have always spawned outbursts of xenophobia. The Black Death of 1348-9 struck a credulous and superstitious European population who sought scapegoats. Some of them blamed themselves, and joined the Brotherhood of the Flagellants, who engaged in self-torture by whipping themselves in frenzied rituals. More generally, the Christian population found scapegoats among the Jews, who were accused of poisoning the wells. In Switzerland, the city of Zürich voted to exclude Jews in perpetuity, while in Basel the Jews were all burnt alive [162][14].

The Covid-19 pandemic has created many opportunities for things that are worse. If even more debt is pushed onto the poor this will only exacerbate the absurdity of the distribution of wealth and stress. We will have to wait until the survivors emerge before we can make any assessment of the incremental psycho-social damage associated with being cut-off from the outside world. There have substantial increases in domestic violence[163] and the psychosocial damage due to isolating vulnerable people will presumably have consequences lasting for a long time.[15] Some technologies being introduced at lightning speed to support Covid-19 interventions, could potentially be repurposed for repression. Like Russia, France released a smartphone app for registering the purpose of movements outside the house, thus giving itself the edge over China in population control, with the technological ability to monitor exactly where phone users are located, and what they are saying, or listening to. I continue to use paper.

The main health impact of the immediate stress and anxiety associated with the epidemic and lockdowns must be to increase levels of chronic disease as discussed in Chapter 3. Adrenaline rushes from intense pressure during epidemics and wars can also have positive aspects some of the time in some people, who over-perform [164]. The West African Ebola epidemic led to new ways of testing and developing vaccines that paid off in the control of subsequent outbreaks [152]. Like a Silicon Valley monopoly Covid-19 has been extraordinarily disruptive[16], moved fast and has broken not just things but people[165].[17] In doing so it is also stimulating innovations not just in biomedicine but also in internet communication. This may lead to long term changes in how people communicate, even delivering on the previously empty promise that video calls will cut down on inefficient and environmentally destructive air travel[18]. This is reminiscent of the innovation hotbeds of the Manhattan Project and Bletchley Park, during World War II, that hatched many of the technologies that underpinned the relatively egalitarian societies that developed afterwards. That is why we have computers that mostly work. This should be a reminder that innovation is not dependent on any one economic model. The future is not constrained to being either one of technological stasis or Silicon Valley's version.

In criticising the mainstream of economics, it is important to remember that in some corners of the world it is a beacon of progress compared with the *status quo*. It is easy to imagine mainstream economics being dismissed as 'the dismal science' in the Trumpian media, as it was by Thomas Carlyle when he coined the phrase in 1849 in a pro-slavery racist tract[167], because they would like to introduce something even worse. The pandemic is hitting hardest in the Anglophone countries where the lies of free-market ideology have been propagated the most. The lies that are exposed by the pandemic do not just include the notion that we need rampant individualist economics to stimulate innovation.

There is also the lie that austerity and strict limits on government budget deficits are sacrosanct. Suddenly massive public expenditure is possible to resolve this crisis. So why was it necessary to impose austerity on the innocent victims of the 2008 crash? The answer can only be found in the mysterious workings of models based on a fantasy world.

The kind of economics that has placed itself at the centre of decision making[19] is founded on a weird perspective, that is fundamentally different from those of other disciplines that engage with the world we live in. It is founded on the philosophy of utilitarianism, which appears reasonable only in a limited set of times and places. It justifies itself with a set of assumptions about human values and psychology that have been repeatedly shown to be wrong. These assumptions are deeply buried in analytical methods that are only accessible to specialists. These methods often seem to evade the critical oversight that is an important part of the experience of those of us who analyse complex phenomena in other fields. They encourage the idea that we can be free of the constraints of nature, hence the dogma of endless economic growth on a finite planet. The pandemic exposes how thin a veneer is this ideology of capitalism. The response to the Covid-19 suggests that the politician who really believes this nonsense is a strawman. That the proponents of the economic theories that depend on it, be they the Rand Foundation or other species on the far right of the political spectrum, are faking belief for the sake of their narrowly defined self-interest. Even establishment figures in the UK starting to question business-as-usual[168]. Especially the myth that all government spending has to be "paid for" is exploded[169].

Mills and Lee[170] wrote in 1993 that we have moved on from the historical focus of health economics being on how to calculate the value of health to the economy, but the idea is still alive in many quarters, especially when there is a possibility of framing an economic evaluation in a self-serving way. Influenced by the vaccine manufacturer, the funders of our first economic evaluation of malaria vaccines [71] wanted us to include among the benefits of malaria vaccination estimates of the increased income of subsistence farmers whose children would no longer fall sick. This is an essentially meaningless quantity (by definition, subsistence agriculture is outside the money economy) but one which would make the vaccine look more valuable than otherwise, and potentially increase subsidies from philanthropy. Similarly, when pharmaceutical companies quote the costs of developing a new drug or vaccine, either to justify the enormous profits they make from licensed pharmaceuticals, they will include as opportunity costs that they forgo by spending money on something of direct benefit rather than investing it on the stock market. But food is cheap, and an increasing proportion of the things we value come with negligible marginal costs (most software, internet use ......). The remainder of what we spend our money on increasingly come under the heading of consumer dross (fashion items, throwaway..... weekends away, the purchase of which becomes stigmatised as the environmental consequences become clear). Investments gain value because of inflated values for art, bubbles in the value of Facebook.......

There is also the lie that state and single payer insurance systems cannot afford to finance the increasing costs of health care(see e.g. [171]). Implicitly, the private sector has an unbounded capacity to grow, and we know that in order to achieve the same level of provision, the private sector grows more (because of the additional transaction costs, profit and rent seeking), with much of the additional employment in Graeber's category of bullshit jobs[172]. Suddenly, however, we find that the state can finance massive scale up of curative care.

Most people would subscribe to the notion that health is a primary good. Inheritance aside, there is no point in being wealthy if you are about to die. As people become richer, they are prepared to spend more on health; as new (and often expensive) technologies are developed there is a demand to use them; and as people live longer, average age and the prevalence of chronic disease increase. The latter is the least important of the three main drivers of cost escalation since the ages at which we become disabled and dependent is also increasing so most of the recent gains in life expectancy are in healthy life-years. All these trends are likely to continue, so health costs will increase. This makes the proportion of expenditure on health seem extraordinarily low, (especially in low income countries), unless there is acknowledgement that it is not only direct health expenditure that improves health.

In Europe, where the necessities of food and clothing have become cheaper and cheaper relative to our incomes, what could be a better way to spend our money than ensuring our health? So, we should be celebrating that we are able to spend more on health, and it is to be expected that more affluent countries have higher health care expenditure. While the quality of life improvements achieved by expenditure in other sectors are often unclear (e.g. the military, fashion, bigger cars) spending on health (i.e. salaries of health workers, medical technologies, pharmaceuticals) generally makes sense. By spending on health, Europeans would seem to be trying to make their lives even better than they have been. Yet perversely, increases in health expenditure are often presented as being bad, unlike general consumption which is thought of as a desirable contribution to the economy, even when the money is being spent on guns or internet scams.

A corollary of the desirability of spending on health is that the more financing of health care is via market mechanisms (or the more choices that are made available), the more the rich spend on it. But they do so inefficiently because it is hard to know which health products are good value. Moreover, the rich tend to be older, and so will spend on high tech therapies close to the end of life, rather than prevention when younger. This may be why the percentage of GDP spent publicly on health services is correlated with life expectancy in OECD countries, but private expenditure on health care is not [164]. We should get used to feeling positive about growing public health care systems.

Beyond the health sector, the economic lies also include the self-serving dogma that vast income inequalities are justified by merit or the need for incentives. This is exposed by the need for some degree of honesty in determining which jobs are non-essential in a lockdown. These include most of the work done by those who self-identify as having useless alienating jobs, described by David Graeber in his viral essay [173] and book [172] as bullshit, which forms a substantial proportion of paid employment. Lockdowns provide a better source of empirical data about the proportion of people in seriously non-essential work, than do the rather unrepresentative surveys carried out by Graeber[172] [20]. The lockdowns make it clearer which are essential services and which people really need to carry on working in a crisis. These are not just the health staff, but also vegetable pickers[21], the garbage collectors, the shelf-stackers, the parcel deliverers. Many of them are people who have been part of the gig economy, paid a pittance, stressed out of their minds, at the same time as being victims of status syndrome. In most countries the teachers, the nurses, and the essential workers who need to carry on working during the pandemic, are paid much less than many of those whose work is totally useless or destructive. Far from this being some strange anomaly, it is exactly what would be expected from research on motivational crowding out [174]. People want to feel they are doing something useful, so health workers and teachers will put up with meagre rewards. On the other hand, if there is no intrinsic motivation because the job is bullshit, then the money is all. Would you work as an advertising executive if it paid the same as a shelf-stacker in a supermarket?[22] If the market really worked then the essential job that nobody really wanted to do (cleaning toilets perhaps) would be paid the most. Market power is a preposterous way of fixing how much people are rewarded for their work, and the notion that redistributive taxation violates some natural law (a commonplace in the USA) is absurd.

Humans strive to achieve all sorts of things, and in our wonderful diversity many of us aim for things that others find incomprehensible or worthless. "Why bother with classical music?" "Why bother eating dark chocolate?" "Why bother watching football?" All these are questions that might seem disrespectful or arrogant, but we can all imagine someone asking them. There are some desires that seem fundamental to the way our societies are constructed; the desire for money, the desire to consume …. To question these might be particularly provocative, but in the liberal democracies of the west we have no difficulty in understanding that not everyone shares these desires.

To call them into question may be unusual but can at least be understood as meaningful. There is something different about asking the question "Why bother with health?" which is rivalled in preposterousness only by questions like "Why bother with sex?". Health has intrinsic value. To question that leads in the direction of madness.

Health is about much more than health care, but buying into the dominant individualistic ideologies, public health interventions in recent years have generally involved trying to discourage people from doing things that are risky. Advocating physical activity and eating lots of fruit and vegetables are about the only positive messaging. Part of what needs to be done is to build societies that think about it less in terms of what we should not do, to what are the things that promote wellbeing [175]. Behavioural economics and nudges have a role to play in this. Not in the sense that they have been applied by advertisers, in their ruthless quest to cream profit via bullshit jobs They have a role because they provide the alternative to a paternalistic or repressive state, and it is not always obvious what makes people's lives better. The insight of Hindman[96], that what works in development is locally specific still applies. Sometimes what works is surprising, and sometimes 'appropriate' technological solutions don't catch on [84]. These insights apply in the industrialised world, as well as where people are poorer.

There has a welcome increase in and recognition of empirical research in economics in recent years, in particular, with the Nobel prize for Banerjee, Duflo and Kremer for their experimental studies of alleviating global poverty in 2019 [176]. The same problem-solving mentality needs to replace the problem creating mentality that still rules most of the western world.

Margaret Thatcher, who said that there is no such thing as society, is dead, but her ghost has continued to haunt the Western world in the form of the rampant individualism and selfishness that has gradually undermined many affluent societies, especially in the Anglophone world, for the last 40 years. But the pandemic-induced epidemic of video connections, shows that even if there can be no physical contact, society is alive. It is deeply ironic that we are forced into a situation where avoiding contact with each other is the best way we can show that we are social beings, that we care for our friends and relatives and for other people we have never met.

Suddenly across Europe, homeless, and migrants who had been cast out on the margins as targets of the hatred of the far-right, are being given shelter because otherwise they would be hotbeds for the spread of the virus. As with the exchange relationships of our primate relatives, or of the Neolithic society of the New Guinea highlands, we can argue endlessly whether this is altruism, or some concealed form of selfishness. We will always be arguing so long as we are alive because we are human.

The lockdowns have led to other strange ironies and eerie echoes and inversions of 20th century history. Paradoxically, the closing of the borders may be bringing us closer together as Europeans. Eighty years ago, we Europeans were killing each other. Today even as the borders are closed, we are finding common cause in saving one another from the Covid-19. This is progress. I have always found Edmund Burke's aphorism that "*Patriotism is the last refuge of a scoundrel*," an obvious truism. I wrote that 8 hours before I was scheduled to video link into a meeting in Bern, where as an Englishman, naturalised as French, I was at a German -speaking meeting to advise the Swiss government on their strategy for the epidemic. Then I returned to the day job of malaria epidemiology, of supporting projects guiding African governments on what to do to avert further epidemics, of malaria, when the ITN delivery programs are disrupted by the Covid-19. There can be no boasting that about managing this. It is just coincidence that it has all come together in the way that it has.

I hope the historians will also look back to the Covid-19 pandemic as the point where money lost its hold on the world, and a new economics and politics took root that is humanist, but that recognises at the same time that we are part of the natural world and inherently limited by it. Let us make sure that our confinement gives birth to a healthy infant. A compassionate world that is ready to face the far greater challenges to come, of the climate emergency that still hangs over us.

---

1   The 'Land of the Unexpected' was the slogan used to promote Papua New Guinean tourism by the national airline in the 1980s, and 'The Small Cosmos' is a book about local variation and quirkiness in many disciplines in New Guinea environments, biology and society. On first encounter with New Guinea, outsiders find this variability and unpredictability strangely disconcerting. There is as much diversity in many of these factors on the island of New Guinea as we find comparing larger areas across the whole world. Now the whole world reminds us that it is not so different from New Guinea.

2   Dramatic transformations of systems can involve predictable tipping points, with gradual build-up to a critical event. Sometimes, as with Covid-19, dramatic events may be just result from an unlikely coincidence of factors, like the asteroid impact that wiped out the dinosaurs. The asteroid that landed in Mexico 60 million years ago was extremely bad luck for some specific populations of Apatosaurus but across the universe asteroid impacts presumably happen continually. There are so many extremely unlikely combinations of events that the probability that none of them happens is vanishingly small. This probability is calculated by multiplying the individual probabilities that each one of them does not happen. Each multiplication of probabilities gives a smaller result, so multiplying many of them gives a tiny number.

3　　The avoidable deaths linked to inequality were presumably just child's play, legitimately sacrificed in a game cooked up on the playing fields of Eton and in the Chicago School of Economics. This is serious, explained his prime minister, widely considered a buffoon, a few days before Covid-19 also caught up with him. Such a moment, when it becomes apparent that what previously appeared to be a game, is not, reminds me of the negotiations of Greek Finance Minister Yanis Varoufakis with the European Central Bank and the European Commission in 2013. Varoufakis tried to exploit his expertise as a game theorist to negotiate cancellation of Greek debt. Unfortunately his opponents were not playing the same game[151]. They did not see it as a game at all. Some of the time, some of the people in power are serious.

4　　A carefully argued article in Wired magazine summarises the rather confusing academic literature on how many people died from the Spanish influenza, concluding this was probably between two and four percent of the global population[152].

5　　I have been on World Health Organisation committees where we discuss the number of people who die each year from malaria, an important statistic that is made much of in the media. An important part of the discussion has been whether the numbers for India are a hundred thousand or so out.

6   This chapter does not consider what is happening in low- and middle-income countries, which raises different issues. At the time of writing, it is not obvious which African and South American countries have large Covid-19 epidemics, but most countries-imposed lockdowns, which may be catastrophic for people who were already living on the edge, with fragile health care systems struggling to cope with other serious infectious diseases.

7   Behavioural economists find that people are more averse to unknown risks that can't be quantified, than to known ones, even if the known risk is of something bad happening with a very high probability[133].

8   In ecology there is the concept of niche exclusion, that two organisms with the same characteristics cannot co-exist. With even a very slight advantage resulting from chance differences between their genomes, one of a pair of near-identical pathogens would inevitably exclude the other. This is a problem both for emergency response, and for outbreak modellers because the specifics of pathogenesis and transmission are initially unknown. Generic models of infectious disease dynamics such as those described in the text of Anderson and May[158], need to be adjusted for each new epidemic organism if they are to prove useful.

There is a whole branch of evolutionary biology that studies the patterns in the ecology of diseases, but ecologists could never have been predicted that a virus with exactly these characteristics would arise. The pandemic illustrates not just the profound uncertainties that we face in modelling epidemic size, but also the general principle that there is a quirkiness in evolution that undermines any certainties about where life is going. The unpredictability of nature leads in turn to unpredictability in historical events.

9   The specialists tasked with answering this question are dealing not only with other people's lives, but with their own futures in academia!

10   Where there is the possibility of rare events such as extinction or seeding of epidemics in specific areas, mathematical models need to allow for randomness (stochasticity) because a model that ignores chance would assume that nothing (or some fraction of an event) would happen..

11   For instance, Tulane University Police Department in New Orleans reported that on April 7, two people were confronted by a gun-toting man who asked if they were Chinese or Japanese, saying, "If you are Chinese or Japanese, I'm going to kill you.".

12   The Swiss psychoanalyst Carl Jung theorised that remarkable coincidences indicate "synchronicity", defined as an "acausal connecting principle", using this to argue that the paranormal exists. Possibly the psychology of this is related to that of conspiracy theories. It may be relevant that Jung had affairs with his patients and was likely permanently stressed.

13   If I suggest to you in advance that when we turn the corner we will encounter a woman wearing pink shoes, a blue dress, a feathered hat, and purple spectacles, you will rightly think that either I have insider information, or that I will almost certainly be wrong. Retrospectively, if having turned the corner we saw her, it is certain we encountered her.

14   My daughter is a schoolteacher in Basel, and I am confident that the Swiss education system has considerably improved since the 14th century, so this kind of thing will not recur here. I have my doubts about other high- income countries that have consistently under-invested in public education.

15   Like a small-scale version of how the blind, maimed, and traumatised victims of WW I haunted western Europe for decades after the Peace of Versailles.

16   It is to be hoped that the word 'disrupt' has now regained its original, negative, connotations. I received a message from the Bill & Melinda Gates Foundation in 2019 announcing that a new kind of toilet for the poor was disrupting sanitation, leading to mental images of broken sewer pipes, and the fear that the sanitation revolution (Chapter 2) might be reversed.

17   Some of the 'players' in Silicon valley have even acknowledged the randomness and destructiveness of much of what they are doing, even labelling themselves as monkeys [166] perhaps as an unconscious reference to the evolutionary pre-history summarised in Chapter 1, though I'm not sure what species they belong to. At least for the moment, during the pandemic, they are caged like the rest of us, though they still roam free in cyberspace.

18   There are downsides of this, since technological innovation disadvantages those who struggle with new technology, who become more and more marginalised. These people need help and support. Many younger people can scarcely imagine that some people struggle to use a mobile phone. There is huge diversity in when in our lives we stop updating with the latest technologies and stick with something we think we understand.

19   Especially in the Anglophone OECD countries, but the European debt crises of the last decade are indicative that the pathology goes much wider. In France we have a president and government which pushes in the same direction.

20   Some categories of bullshit, notably cold calling, seem to have been especially hard hit.

21   For instance, In Alsace there was recruiting of non-essential workers to pick the asparagus crop usually harvested by eastern Europeans, cut-off by the lockdown. Those normally condemned to bullshit jobs[173] are getting their hands dirty.

22   *"If paying someone to work reduces motivation, then top executives who get paid millions actually do nothing. Nobody is saying that though, even if billionaires aren't motivated to do anything, they can afford lawyers who are."* —Burnett[17]

References

[1]   T. JEFFERSON and C. HENEGHAN. "Modelling the Models." CEBM. https://www.cebm.net/2020/04/modelling-the-models (accessed 5 April, 2020).

[2]   A. H. MASLOW, *Motivation and personality*, 3rd ed. ed. Harper and Row, 1987.

[3]   T. HOBBES, *Leviathan*. London: Andrew Crooke, 1651.

[4]   J.-J. ROUSSEAU, *Du contrat social, ou, Principes du droit politique et autres écrits autour du Contrat social*. Amsterdam: Marc-Michel Rey 1762.

[5]   M. MARMOT, *Status syndrome : how your social standing directly affects your health and life expectancy*. London: Bloomsbury, 2004.

[6]   R. G. WILKINSON and K. PICKETT, *The spirit level : why equality is better for everyone*. London: Penguin, 2010.

[7]   PLATO and H. D. P. LEE, *The Republic*, 2nd edition (revised). ed. (Penguin classics). Harmondsworth ; Baltimore: Penguin, 1974.

[8]   S. GEMAN and D. GEMAN, "Stochastic Relaxation, Gibbs Distributions, and the Bayesian Restoration of Images," *IEEE Transactions on Pattern Analysis and Machine Intelligence (Volume: , Issue: 6 , Nov. 1984)* vol. PAMI-6, no. 6, pp. 721 - 741,1984

[9]   Y. N. HARARI, *Sapiens : a brief history of humankind*, First U.S. edition. ed. New York: Harper, 2015.

[10]   S. BHATT *et al.*, "The effect of malaria control on Plasmodium falciparum in Africa between 2000 and 2015," *Nature,* vol. 526, no. 7572, pp. 207-+,2015

[11]   M. L. PAGE. Can we really save the planet by making food 'from air' without farms? *New Scientist*. (10 January 2020)

[12]   N. N. TALEB, *The black swan : the impact of the highly improbable*. London: Allen Lane, 2007.

[13]   L. GARRETT, *The coming plague : newly emerging diseases in a world out of balance*. New York: Farrar, Straus and Giroux, 1994.

[14]   WORLD HEALTH ORGANISATION. "Global Health Expenditure Database." https://apps.who.int/nha/database/ViewData/Indicators/en (accessed April 2, 2020).

[15]   W. STORR, *The science of storytelling*. Collins, 2019.

[16]   R. H. TAWNEY, *Religion and the Rise of Capitalism : A Historical Study*. West Drayton: Pelican Books, 1926.

[17]   D. BURNETT, *The idiot brain : a neuroscientist explains what your head is really up to*. New York: Norton, 2016.

[18]   S. SCOTT and C. J. DUNCAN, *Biology of plagues : evidence from historical populations*. Cambridge: Cambridge University Press, 2001.

[19]   M. SAHLINS, *Stone Age economics*. London: Tavistock Publications, 1974.

[20]   E. J. EYRE, *Journals of Expeditions of discovery into Central Australia, and overland from Adelaide to King George's Sound, in 1840-1, including an account of the manners and customs of the Aborigines, and the state of their relations with Europeans*. London :: T. and W. Boone, 1845.

[21]   A. SMITH, *An inquiry into the nature and causes of the wealth of nations*. London: Straman, 1776.

[22]   D. GRAEBER, *Debt : the first 5,000 years*. New York: Melville House, 2011.

[23]   J. M. DIAMOND, *The world until yesterday : what can we learn from traditional societies?* London: Allen Lane, 2012.

[24]   C. L. JENKINS, "Health in the early contact period: a contemporary example from Papua New Guinea," *Soc Sci Med,* vol. 26, no. 10, pp. 997-1006,1988

[25]   A. DEATON, *The Great Escape: health, wealth and the origins of inequality*. Princeton,N.J.: Princeton University Press, 2013.

[26] M. MAUSS, *The gift : Forms and functions of exchange on Archaic Societies*. London: Cohen & West, 1969.

[27] R. I. M. DUNBAR, "Coevolution of neocortical size, group size and language in humans," *Behavioral and Brain Sciences,* vol. 16, no. 4, pp. 681-694,1993

[28] J. GUIART, "John Frum Movement in Tanna," *Oceania,* vol. 22, 3, pp. 165-177,1952

[29] D. MILLER, *Unwrapping Christmas*. Oxford: Clarendon Press, 1993.

[30] B. M. FAGAN, *Floods, famines and emperors : El Niño and the fate of civilizations*. London: Pimlico, 1999.

[31] J. C. SCOTT, *Against the grain : a deep history of the earliest states*. New Haven and London: Yale University Press, 2017.

[32] W. H. MCNEILL, *Plagues and peoples*, 1st ed. ed. Garden City, N.Y.: Anchor Press, 1976.

[33] J. LANCHESTER, *Whoops! : why everyone owes everyone and no one can pay*. London: Penguin, 2010.

[34] W. SCHEIDEL, *The Great Leveler: Violence and the History of Inequality from the Stone Age to the Twenty-First Century*. New York: Princeton University Press, 2017.

[35] P. H. WILSON, *Europe's tragedy : a history of the Thirty Years War*. London: Allen Lane, 2009.

[36] GAPMINDER. "Gapminder." https://www.gapminder.org (accessed 6 April 2020.

[37] E. A. WRIGLEY and R. S. SCHOFIELD, *The Population History of England 1541–1871*. Cambridge: Cambridge University Press, 1989.

[38] T. H. HOLLINGSWORTH, *The Demography of the British peerage*. London: London School of Economics, 1964.

[39] E. P. THOMPSON, *Making of the English Working Class*. [S.l.]: V.Gollancz, 1963.

[40] H. RITCHIE and M. ROSER. "Urbanization." https://ourworldindata.org/urbanization#urban-slum-populations (accessed 1 May 2020.

[41]   R. W. FOGEL, *The Escape from Hunger and Premature Death, 1700-2100*. Cambridge: Cambridge University Press, 2004.

[42]   WORLD HEALTH ORGANISATION, "Global Eradication of Smallpox: Final Report of the Global Commission for the Certification of Smallpox Eradication," World Health Organisation, Geneva, 1979.

[43]   D. A. HENDERSON, *Smallpox: The Death of a Disease - The Inside Story of Eradicating a Worldwide Killer*. Amherst, New York, USA: Prometheus Books, 2009.

[44]   F. PACINI, "Osservazioni microscopiche e deduzioni patologiche sul cholera asiatico " *Gazzetta Medica Italiana: Toscana. 2nd series,*, vol. 4, no. 51, pp. 405-412,1854

[45]   INDEPTH NETWORK, *Measuring Health Equity in Small Areas: Findings from Demographic Surveillance Systems*. Farnham: Ashworth, 2005.

[46]   M. C. NUSSBAUM and A. SEN, *Quality of Life*. Oxford: Oxford University Press, 1993.

[47]   T. MCKEOWN, *The Role of Medicine: Dream, mirage or nemesis?* London: Nuffield Trust, 1976.

[48]   D. BLACK, J. N. MORRIS, C. SMITH, P. TOWNSEND, and M. WHITEHEAD, *The Black Report & The Health Divide*. Pelican 1988.

[49]   M. BARTLEY, *Health Inequality*. Cambridge: Polity Press, 2004.

[50]   M. A. MARMOT, *The health gap : the challenge of an unequal world*. Bloomsbury Publishing 2016.

[51]   J. O. JONSSON and C. MILLS, *Cradle to grave : life-course change in modern Sweden*. Durham: Sociology Press, 2001.

[52]   R. G. A. WILKINSON and K. A. PICKETT, *The inner level : how more equal societies reduce stress, restore sanity and improve everybody's wellbeing*. Penguin, 2019.

[53]   C. J. L. MURRAY *et al.*, "Disability-adjusted life years (DALYs) for 291 diseases and injuries in 21 regions,

1990ΓÇô2010: a systematic analysis for the Global Burden of Disease Study 2010," *The Lancet,* vol. 380, no. 9859, pp. 2197-2223,2012

[54] E. DURKHEIM, *Le Suicide. étude de sociologie.* Paris: Germer Ballière, 1897.

[55] H. MANTEL, *Wolf Hall,* Large print ed. ed. [Bath]: Windsor, 2010, 2009.

[56] F. FUKUYAMA, *The end of history and the last man.* London: Hamilton, 1992.

[57] E. J. HOBSBAWM, *Age of extremes : the short twentieth century, 1914-1991.* London: Abacus, 1995.

[58] T. PIKETTY, *Capital in the Twenty-First Century.* Cambridge, MS: Harvard University Press, 2014.

[59] B. MILANOVIC, *Global inequality : a new approach for the age of globalization.* Boston: Harvard University Press, 2016.

[60] ORGANISATION FOR ECONOMIC CO-OPERATION AND DEVELOPMENT. "OECD data." https://data.oecd.org/ (accessed 6 April 2020.

[61] D. KAHNEMAN, *Thinking, fast and slow.* London: Penguin, 2012.

[62] T. SMITH *et al.*, "Mathematical modeling of the impact of malaria vaccines on the clinical epidemiology and natural history of plasmodium Falciparum malaria: Overview," *Am J Trop Med Hyg,* vol. 75, no. 2, pp. 1-10,2006

[63] T. SMITH *et al.*, "Towards a comprehensive simulation model of malaria epidemiology and control," *Parasitology,* vol. 135, no. 13, pp. 1507-1516,2008

[64] T. SMITH *et al.*, "Relationships between the entomological inoculation rate and the force of infection for *Plasmodium falciparum* malaria," *Am J Trop Med Hyg,* vol. 75 (Suppl 2), pp. 11-18,2006

[65] T. SMITH, G. KILLEEN, C. LENGELER, and M. TANNER, "Relationships between the outcome of *Plasmodium falciparum* infection and the intensity of transmission in

Africa," *Am J Trop Med Hyg,* vol. 71 (2 Suppl), no. 2 Suppl, pp. 80-86,2004

[66] M. E. WOOLHOUSE *et al.,* "Heterogeneities in the transmission of infectious agents: implications for the design of control programs," *Proc Natl Acad Sci USA,* vol. 94, no. 1, pp. 338-342,1997

[67] T. A. SMITH, "Estimation of heterogeneity in malaria transmission by stochastic modelling of apparent deviations from mass action kinetics," *Malaria J,* vol. 7,2008

[68] T. SMITH *et al.,* "Ensemble Modeling of the Likely Public Health Impact of a Pre- Erythrocytic Malaria Vaccine," *Plos Med,* vol. 9, no. 1,2012

[69] D. KAHNEMAN and A. TVERSKY, "Prospect Theory - Analysis of Decision under Risk," *Econometrica,* vol. 47, no. 2, pp. 263-291,1979

[70] F. ENGELS, *Condition of the Working Class in England.* Panther, 1969.

[71] F. TEDIOSI, G. HUTTON, N. MAIRE, T. A. SMITH, A. ROSS, and M. TANNER, "Predicting the cost-effectiveness of introducing a pre-erythrocytic malaria vaccine into the expanded program on immunization in Tanzania," *Am J Trop Med Hyg,* vol. 75, no. 2, pp. 131-143,2006

[72] F. TEDIOSI, N. MAIRE, M. A. PENNY, A. STUDER, and T. A. SMITH, "Simulation of the cost-effectiveness of malaria vaccines," *Malar. J,* vol. 8, p. 127,2009

[73] WORLD HEALTH ORGANISATION. Malaria vaccine: WHO position paper – January 2016. *Weekly epidemiological record.* 33–52 (29 Jan 2016)

[74] C. DICKENS, *David Copperfield.* London: Bradbury & Evans, 1850.

[75] J. HANLON, A. BARRIENTOS, and D. HULME, *Just give money to the poor : the development revolution from the global south.* Sterling, VA: Kumarian Press, 2010.

[76]   J. RIFKIN, *The end of work : the decline of the global labor force and the dawn of the post-market era*. New York: G.P. Putnam's Sons, 1995.

[77]   W. KENTON. "Shock Therapy." https://www.investopedia.com/terms/s/shock-therapy.asp (accessed 16 April 2020, 2020).

[78]   J. SACHS, "The Bolivian Hyperinflation and Stabilization," *AEA Papers and Proceedings*, vol. 77, no. 2, pp. 279-283,1987

[79]   J. TELFORD. "Che Guevara and the Price of Toilet Paper." https://julietee.wordpress.com/2011/02/21/che-guevara-and-the-price-of-toilet-paper/ (accessed.

[80]   WORLD BANK. "World Bank Open Data." https://data.worldbank.org (accessed 6 April 2020.

[81]   F. BLACK and M. SCHOLES, "The Pricing of Options and Corporate Liabilities," *Journal of Political Economy*, vol. 81, 3, pp. 637-654,1973

[82]   J. H. VINCENT, D. C. STEVENS, D. MARK, M. MARSHALL, and T. A. SMITH, "On the Aspiration Characteristics of Large-Diameter, Thin-Walled Aerosol Sampling Probes at Yaw Orientations with Respect to the Wind," *J Aerosol Sci*, vol. 17, no. 2, pp. 211-&,1986

[83]   D. H. MEADOWS, D. L. MEADOWS, J. RANDERS, and W. W. BEHRENS, *The limits to growth : A report for the Club of Rome's project on The Predicament of Mankind*. New York: A Potomac Associates Book, 1972.

[84]   A. V. BANERJEE and E. DUFLO, *Good Economics for Hard Times : Better Answers to Our Biggest Problems*. Penguin Random House UK, 2019.

[85]   W. BANK, "Investing in Health," in "World Development Report," Oxford, 1993 1993.

[86]   J. L. GALLUP and J. SACHS, "The economic burden of malaria," *Am J Trop Med Hyg*, vol. 64, no. 1-2 Suppl, pp. 85-96,2001

[87]   N. SARMA, E. PATOUILLARD, R. E. CIBULSKIS, and J.-L. ARCAND, "The Economic Burden of Malaria: Revisiting

the Evidence," *The American Journal of Tropical Medicine and Hygiene,* vol. 101, no. 6, pp. 1405-1415,2019

[88]   J. WILSON, *Jeffrey Sachs : the strange case of Dr Shock and Mr Aid.* London ; New York: Verso, 2014.

[89]   S. J. WANG *et al.,* "Rapid Urban Malaria Appraisal (RUMA) II: epidemiology of urban malaria in Dar es Salaam (Tanzania)," *Malar J,* vol. 5, p. 28,2006

[90]   WORLD BANK, "Investing in Health," in "World Development Report," Oxford, 1993.

[91]   GFATM. "The Global Fund to Fight AIDS, Tuberculosis and Malaria." https://www.theglobalfund.org/en/overview/ (accessed 12 April 2020, 2020).

[92]   GAVI. "Gavi, the Vaccine Alliance." https://www.gavi.org/our-alliance/about (accessed 12 April 2020, 2020).

[93]   P. K. PIFF, D. M. STANCATO, S. CÔTÉ, R. MENDOZA-DENTON, and D. KELTNER, "Higher social class predicts increased unethical behavior," *Proceedings of the National Academy of Sciences,* vol. 109, no. 11, pp. 4086-4091,2012

[94]   R. SUGDEN, "On the Economics of Philanthropy," *The Economic Journal,* vol. 92, no. 366, pp. 341-350,1982

[95]   B. ELTON, *This other Eden.* London: Pocket Books, 1993.

[96]   A. HIRSHMAN, "Political Economics and Possibilism," in *A Bias for Hope: Essays on Development in Latin America*: Yale University Press, 1971, pp. 1-34.

[97]   HERODOTUS, *The Histories.* Penguin, 1996.

[98]   W. MACASKILL, *Doing good better : how effective altruism can help you make a difference.* Random House, 2015.

[99]   R. ROSS, "On some peculiar pigmented cells found in two mosquitoes fed on malarial blood.," *BMJ,* vol. ii, pp. 1786-1788,1897

[100] G. G. and P. F. BEALES, "The recent history of malaria control and eradication.," in *Malaria, Principles and Practice of Malariology*, W. H. Wernsdorfer and I. Mc Gregor Eds. Edinburgh: Churchill Livingstone, 1988, ch. 45, pp. 1335-1378.

[101] G. MACDONALD, "Theory of the eradication of malaria," *Bull World Health Org*, no. 15, pp. 369-87,1956

[102] R. SNOW, K. M. ROWAN, and B. M. GREENWOOD, "A trial of permethrin-treated bed nets in the prevention of malaria in Gambian children," *Trans R Soc Trop Med & Hyg*, vol. 81, no. 4, pp. 563-567,1987

[103] S. W. LINDSAY, R. SNOW, G. L. BROOMFIELD, M. S. JANNEH, R. A. WIRTZ, and B. M. GREENWOOD, "Impact of permethrin-treated bednets on malaria transmission by the *Anopheles gambiae* complex in The Gambia," *Med Vet Entomol*, vol. 3, no. 3, pp. 263-271,1989

[104] P. L. ALONSO *et al.*, "The effect of insecticide-treated bed nets on mortality of Gambian children," *Lancet*, vol. 337, no. 8756, pp. 1499-1502,1991

[105] D. STÜRCHLER, "How much malaria is there in the world?," *Parasitology Today*, vol. 5, pp. 39-40,1989

[106] F. BINKA *et al.*, "Impact of permethrin impregnated bednets on child mortality in Kassena-Nankana district, Ghana: a randomized controlled trial," *Trop Med Int Health*, vol. 1, no. 2, pp. 147-154,1996

[107] C. NEVILL *et al.*, "Insecticide-treated bednets reduce mortality and severe morbidity from malaria among children on the Kenyan coast," *Trop Med Int Health*, vol. 1, no. 2, pp. 139-146,1996

[108] P. PHILLIPS-HOWARD *et al.*, "Efficacy of permethrin-treated bed nets in the prevention of mortality in young children in an area of high perennial malaria transmission in western Kenya," *Am J Trop Med Hyg*, vol. 68 (Suppl. 4), pp. 23-29,2003

[109] C. LENGELER, "Insecticide-treated bed nets and curtains for preventing malaria," *Cochrane. Database. Syst. Rev,* no. 2, p. CD000363,2004

[110] K. HANSON *et al.,* "Cost-effectiveness of social marketing of insecticide-treated nets for malaria control in the United Republic of Tanzania," *Bull World Health Organ,* vol. 81, no. 4, pp. 269-76,2003

[111] J. R. ARMSTRONG SCHELLENBERG *et al.,* "KINET: a social marketing programme of treated nets and net treatment for malaria control in Tanzania, with evaluation of child health and long-term survival," *Trans R Soc Trop Med Hyg,* vol. 93, pp. 225-231,1999

[112] K. A. LINDBLADE *et al.,* "Evaluation of long-lasting insecticidal nets after 2 years of household use," *Trop. Med. Int. Health,* vol. 10, no. 11, pp. 1141-1150,2005

[113] S. M. MAGESA *et al.,* "Trial of pyrethroid impregnated bednets in an area of Tanzania holoendemic for malaria. Part 2. Effects on the malaria vector population," *Acta Trop,* vol. 49, no. 2, pp. 97-108,1991

[114] R. SNOW and K. MARSH, "Will reducing *Plasmodium falciparum* transmission alter malaria mortality among African children?," *Parasitol Today,* vol. 11, no. 5, pp. 188-190,1995

[115] F. BINKA, F. INDOME, and T. SMITH, "Impact of spatial distribution of permethrin-impregnated bed nets on child mortality in rural northern Ghana," *Am J Trop Med Hyg,* vol. 59, no. 1, pp. 80-85,1998

[116] W. A. HAWLEY *et al.,* "Community-Wide effects of Permethrin-treated bed nets on child mortality and malaria morbidiy in Western Kenya," *Am J Trop Med Hyg,* vol. 68 (Suppl. 4), pp. 121-127,2003

[117] G. F. KILLEEN *et al.,* "Quantifying behavioural interactions between humans and mosquitoes: Evaluating the protective efficacy of insecticidal nets against malaria transmission in rural Tanzania," *Bmc Infect Dis,* vol. 6,2006

[118] A. R. SEXTON, "Best practices for an insecticide-treated bed net distribution programme in sub-Saharan eastern Africa," *Malaria J,* vol. 10, no. 1, p. 157,2011

[119] ROLL BACK MALARIA, WORLD HEALTH ORGANISATION, and UNICEF, *World Malaria Report 2005.* Geneva: WHO and UNICEF, 2005.

[120] WORLD HEALTH ORGANISATION, "World Malaria Report 2019," Geneva, 2020.

[121] W. EASTERLY, *The tyranny of experts : economists, dictators, and the forgotten rights of the poor.* New York: Basic Books, a member of the Perseus Book Group, 2013.

[122] P. COLLIER, *The bottom billion : why the poorest countries are failing and what can be done about it.* Oxford: Oxford University Press, 2007.

[123] M. RUNGE *et al.,* "Simulating the council-specific impact of anti-malaria interventions: A tool to support malaria strategic planning in Tanzania," *Plos One,* vol. 15, no. 2, p. e0228469,2020

[124] C. J. L. MURRAY and A. D. LOPEZ, *The global burden of disease: a comprehensive assessment of mortality and disability from diseases, injuries, and risk factors in 1990 and projected to 2020.* Boston: Harvard University Press, 1996.

[125] J. BRAZIER, "Valuing Health States for Use in Cost-Effectiveness Analysis," *PharmacoEconomics,* vol. 26, no. 9, pp. 769-779,2008

[126] M. F. DRUMMOND, B. J. O`BRIEN, G. L. STODDART, and G. W. TORRANCE, *Methods for the economic evaluation of health care programmes,* 2 ed. Oxford: Oxford Medical Publications, 1998.

[127] J. RAWLS, *A theory of justice.* Oxford: Clarendon Press, 1972.

[128] K. ARROW, "A Difficulty in the Concept of Social Welfare," *Journal of Political Economy,* vol. 58, no. 4, pp. 328-346,1950

[129]   A. J. CULYER, *Encyclopedia of health economics*. Elsevier 2014.

[130]   J. J. THOMSON, *The Trolley Problem/ Das Trolley-Problem* (Reclams Universal-Bibliothek, no. 19658). 1985.

[131]   F. R. JOHNSON, M. R. BANZHAF, and W. H. DESVOUSGES, "Willingness to pay for improved respiratory and cardiovascular health: a multiple-format, stated-preference approach," *Health Econ,* vol. 9, no. 4, pp. 295-317,2000

[132]   J. E. H. SMITH, *Irrationality: A History of the Dark Side of Reason*. Princeton: Princeton University Pres, 2019.

[133]   E. CARTWRIGHT, *Behavioral economics*, Third edition. ed. Routledge, 2018.

[134]   B. MCPAKE, L. KUMARANAYAKE, and C. NORMAND, *Health economics : an international perspective*. London: Routledge, 2002.

[135]   R. A. HIRTH, M. E. CHERNEW, and E. MILLER, "Willingness to Pay for a Quality-adjusted Life Year: In Search of a Standard," *Medical Decision Making,* vol. 20, no. 3, pp. 332-42,2000

[136]   A. SEN, *Behaviour and the concept of preference. (An inaugural lecture.)*. [London]: London School of Economics and Political Science, 1973.

[137]   A. SEN, *Maximization and the act of choice*. Rome: Banca D' Italia, 1996.

[138]   A. SEN, *Rationality and freedom*. Cambridge, Mass. ; London: Belknap Press, 2002.

[139]   R. M. TITMUSS, *The gift relationship : from human blood to social policy*. London: Allen & Unwin, 1970.

[140]   C. MCCABE, K. CLAXTON, and A. J. CULYER, "The NICE Cost-Effectiveness Threshold," *PharmacoEconomics,* vol. 26, no. 9, pp. 733-744,2008

[141]   B. WOODS, P. REVILL, M. SCULPHER, and K. CLAXTON, "Country-Level Cost-Effectiveness Thresholds: Initial

Estimates and the Need for Further Research," *Value Health,* vol. 19, no. 8, pp. 929-935,2016

[142] N. KUNZLI *et al.,* "Public-health impact of outdoor and traffic-related air pollution: a European assessment," *Lancet,* vol. 356, no. 9232, pp. 795-801,2000

[143] P. N. SKANDALAKIS, P. LAINAS, O. ZORAS, J. E. SKANDALAKIS, and P. MIRILAS, ""To afford the wounded speedy assistance": Dominique Jean Larrey and Napoleon," *World J Surg,* vol. 30, no. 8, pp. 1392-9,2006

[144] SWISS ACADEMY OF MEDICAL SCIENCES, "COVID-19 pandemic: triage for intensive-care treatment under resource scarcity," *Swiss Med Wkly. ,* vol. 150, p. w20229,2020

[145] UNITED NATIONS DEVELOPMENT PROGRAM. "Human Development Index." http://hdr.undp.org/en/content/human-development-index-hdi (accessed 21 April 2020, 2020).

[146] G. BEVAN and C. HOOD, "Have targets improved performance in the English NHS?," *BMJ,* vol. 332, no. 7538, pp. 419-422,2006

[147] I. FINLAY, "UK strategies for palliative care," *J R Soc Med,* vol. 94, no. 9, pp. 437-441,2001

[148] W. WORDSWORTH. "The Prelude " https://romantic-circles.org/editions/poets/texts/preludeXII.html (accessed 21 April 2020, 2020).

[149] G. MONBIOT, *Feral : rewilding the land, the sea, and human life.* Penguin, 2013.

[150] R. DAWKINS, *The selfish gene.* Oxford: Oxford University Press, 1976.

[151] Y. VAROUFAKIS, *Adults in the room : my battle with Europe's deep establishment.* Farrar Strauss & Giroux 2017.

[152] F. JABR. Covid-19 Is Not the Spanish Flu. *Wired.* (13 March 2020).Available: https://www.wired.com/story/covid-19-is-nothing-like-the-spanish-flu/

[153]   S. HEHLI and A. NIEDERER, "Experte zum Corona-Ausbruch: «Man muss jetzt nicht die halbe Schweiz unter Quarantäne stellen," in *Neue Zürcher Zeitung*, ed. Zürich, 2020.

[154]   A. RODRIGUEZ, "Texas' lieutenant governor suggests grandparents are willing to die for US economy," in *USA Today*, ed, 2020.

[155]   M. S. DANIEL MEIER, "Wie viel Geld darf ein Menschenleben kosten? Die heikle Frage in der Corona-Krise," in *Neue Zürcher Zeitung*, ed. Zürich, 2020.

[156]   A. O. D. BERKER *et al.*, "Computations of uncertainty mediate acute stress responses in humans," *Nature Communications,* vol. 7, p. 10996,2015

[157]   W. O. KERMACK and A. G. MCKENDRICK, "Contributions to the mathematical theory of epidemics--I," *Proc Roy Soc A,* vol. 115, no. 772, pp. 700-721,1927

[158]   R. M. ANDERSON and R. M. MAY, *Infectious Diseases of Humans: Dynamics and Control.* Oxford: Oxford University Press, 1991.

[159]   J. E. USCINSKI and J. M. PARENT, *American conspiracy theories.* Oxford ; New York: Oxford University Press, 2014.

[160]   UNAIDS. "Global HIV & AIDS statistics — 2019 fact sheet." UNAIDS. https://www.unaids.org/en/resources/fact-sheet (accessed 10 April 2020, 2020).

[161]   P. OLTERMANN *et al.*, "The cluster effect: how social gatherings were rocket fuel for coronavirus," in *The Guardian*, ed. London: Guardian Newspapers, 2020.

[162]   P. ZIEGLER, *The black death*. Stroud: Sutton, 1997, 1969.

[163]   A. TAUB, "A New Covid-19 Crisis: Domestic Abuse Rises Worldwide," in *New York Times*, ed. New York, 2020.

[164]   H. THOMSON. Don't stress: The scientific secrets of people who keep cool heads. *New Scientist*. (19 February 2020)

[165] J. T. TAPLIN, *Move fast and break things : how Facebook, Google, and Amazon have cornered culture and what it means for all of us*. Macmillan, 2017.

[166] A. GARCÌA MARTÌNEZ, *Chaos monkeys : inside the Silicon Valley money machine*. HarperCollins, 2016.

[167] T. CARLYLE. Occasional Discourse on the Negro Question. *Fraser's Magazine for Town and Country*. 670–679 (December 1849)

[168] M. CARNEY. By invitation: Mark Carney on how the economy must yield to human values. *The Economist*. (Apr16 2020)

[169] Y. NERSISYAN and L. R. WRAY, "Coronavirus has destroyed the myth of the deficit," in *The Guardian*, ed. London: Guardian Newspapers, 2020.

[170] A. MILLS and K. LEE, *Health Economics Research in Developing Countries*. Oxford: Oxford University Press, 1993.

[171] R. G. EVANS, "Illusions of necessity: evading responsibility for choice in health care," *J Health Polit Policy Law,* vol. 10, no. 3, pp. 439-67,1985

[172] D. GRAEBER, *Bullshit jobs : a theory*. Allen Lane, 2018.

[173] D. GRAEBER. On the Phenomenon of Bullshit Jobs: A Work Rant. *Strike*. (August 2013)

[174] B. S. FREY and R. JEGEN, "Motivation crowding theory," *J Econ Surv,* vol. 15, no. 5, pp. 589-611,2001

[175] P. HANLON, S. CARLISLE, M. HANNAH, D. REILLY, and A. LYON, "Making the case for a 'fifth wave' in public health," *Public Health,* vol. 125, no. 1, pp. 30-36,2011

[176] THE ROYAL SWEDISH ACADEMY OF SCIENCES, "Press release: The Prize in Economic Sciences 2019," ed. Stockholm, 2019.

CPSIA information can be obtained
at www.ICGtesting.com
Printed in the USA
LVHW030127210421
685088LV00001B/45